The Athletic Woman's Survival Guide

How to win the battle against eating disorders, amenorrhea, and osteoporosis

Carol L. Otis, MD, FACSM
Roger Goldingay

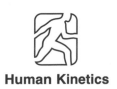

Human Kinetics

Library of Congress Cataloging-in-Publication Data

Otis, Carol L.
   The athletic woman's survival guide: how to win the battle against eating disorders, amenorrhea, and osteoporosis/Carol L. Otis, Roger Goldingay.
      p. cm.
   Includes bibliographical references and index.
   ISBN: 0-7360-0121-2
   1. Women athletes--Health and hygiene. 2. Women athletes--Diseases. 3. Eating disorders. 4. Amenorrhea. 5. Osteoporosis in women. I. Goldingay, Roger. II. Title.

   RC1218.W65 O68 2000
   617.1'027'082--dc21   99-055550

ISBN: 0-7360-0121-2

Developmental Editor: Julie Rhoda; **Assistant Editor:** Carla Zych; **Copyeditor:** Lisa Morgan; **Proofreader:** Joanna Hatzopoulos; **Indexer:** Nan N. Badgett; **Graphic Designer:** Fred Starbird; **Graphic Artist:** Dody Bullerman; **Photo Editor:** Clark Brooks; **Cover Designer:** Jack W. Davis; **Photographer (cover):** D. Graham/H. Armstrong Roberts; **Photographers (interior):** Photos on pp. 24, 41, 54, 86, and 145 by Tom Roberts; **Illustrator:** Tom Roberts; **Printer:** United Graphics

Human Kinetics books are available at special discounts for bulk purchase. Special editions or book excerpts can also be created to specification. For details, contact the Special Sales Manager at Human Kinetics.

Printed in the United States of America   10   9   8   7   6   5   4   3   2   1

Human Kinetics
Web site: **www.humankinetics.com**

United States: Human Kinetics
P.O. Box 5076
Champaign, IL 61825-5076
800-747-4457
e-mail: humank@hkusa.com

Canada: Human Kinetics
475 Devonshire Road Unit 100
Windsor, ON N8Y 2L5
800-465-7301 (in Canada only)
e-mail: hkcan@mnsi.net

Europe: Human Kinetics, P.O. Box IW14
Leeds LS16 6TR, United Kingdom
+44 (0)113-278 1708
e-mail: humank@hkeurope.com

Australia: Human Kinetics
57A Price Avenue
Lower Mitcham, South Australia 5062
08 8277 1555
e-mail: liahka@senet.com.au

New Zealand: Human Kinetics
P.O. Box 105-231, Auckland Central
09-309-1890
e-mail: hkp@ihug.co.nz

This book is dedicated to women—in all their wonderful shapes, sizes, and colors.

Contents

Foreword

Women, especially female athletes, have always been judged by their appearance. I'll never forget the time I was told by a good friend and supporter, "You'll be good because you're ugly, Billie Jean." I was 16 at the time, and this comment was devastating. It is the kind of comment, stated in a friendly, offhanded way, that can shatter the confidence of a young woman. It's similar to, "If you just lost a few pounds, you'd be a better runner, swimmer, jumper, tennis player . . . take your pick." It's the kind of comment that can kick off a frenzied attempt to please, to lose a few pounds, to do *something* to make yourself more attractive, faster, or better. We women will bend over backward to please our critics, despite their thoughtless, inconsiderate, and totally unfounded comments.

What I love about *The Athletic Woman's Survival Guide* is that it lays out all the reasons to ignore the critics and it helps us refute the misguided attempts to change us in impossible and health-threatening ways. Here we can learn to recognize the subtle and insidious ways the media, advertising, and society in general try to make us want to be someone we are not, and in fact can *never* be. The health risks and damage to our performance and self-esteem can be enormous—even life threatening.

The Athletic Woman's Survival Guide doesn't just say the critics are wrong; this book also points out how their comments are not based in any kind of science. Dr. Carol Otis and Roger Goldingay give us real tools to deal with these situations and they teach us how to know ourselves. You will learn how to tell if you really are overweight or overtraining and what to do about it. You will also learn how to deal with those people who have power in our lives, such as coaches, parents, teammates, and trainers.

This is a practical book, one I wish I had had long ago. It could have saved me many years of struggling with diet and weight issues and trying to find myself in a world that always seemed to want me to be something else. Read *The Athletic Woman's Survival Guide* for yourself, and then pass it on to a friend. Get the word out to the young generation of women who now have opportunities to participate that were not available 20 or even 10 years ago. Let's make sport and exercise the wonderful, empowering activity we know it can be for all women.

Billie Jean King
May 8, 2000

Acknowledgments

Many wonderful people assisted in the vision, creation, and production of this book. We would like to thank everyone who helped us, including all the athletes, friends, and supporters who made it possible by sharing their problems and solutions. There are so many people to thank that we would surely miss half of them if we tried to list them all.

In the beginning were the women who shared their stories with us and taught us about the female athlete triad before it was defined. In those early days, Carol's colleagues at UCLA and ACSM helped us understand these perplexing disorders. Special thanks to Barbara Drinkwater, PhD, the inspiring voice, dedicated researcher, and role model. She challenged us to do the work and to raise awareness about the female athlete triad.

Many thanks to Rosemary Agostini, MD; Sheri Albert, MPH, RD; Harmon Brown, MD; Barbara Campaign, PhD; Sara Cates; Michael Dobie; Joani Essenmacher, ATC, PT; Glenn Gaesser, PhD; Barb Harris; Robert Hatcher, MD; Pat Henry; Mimi Johnson, MD; Ben Kibler, MD; Billie Jean King; Felice Kurtzman, MPH, RD; MD; Gerry Lahanas; Connie LeBrun, MD; Donna Lopiano, PhD; Judy Lutter; Lyle Micheli, MD; Steve Park; Paul Roetert, PhD; Randa Ryan, PhD; Barney Sanborn, PhD; Pete Sinclair; Kathleen Stroia, ATC, PT; Christine Snow, PhD; Michelle Warren, MD; and Jack Wilmore, PhD.

Special appreciation to our editor, Julie Rhoda, who kept us on course through title changes and photo searches and streamlined our thoughts and words into coherent chapters. And thank you, Rainer Martens, for believing in us and getting the word out about the female athlete triad.

Introduction

Shannon grew up playing sports with her brothers. She played basketball and soccer in high school and loved swimming with her club team. She felt her best being strong and muscular and said she liked the way she looked because she knew she was in great shape. She never weighed herself and ate pretty much whatever she wanted. She knew of girls who dieted all the time, and she would say, "That's stupid. Diet is definitely the wrong word around our house. Playing sports is more important to me than looking a certain way. I can eat all I want and never gain weight because I like to work out. I have fun, and I have way more confidence in myself than those girls who are always dieting."

Leah was the best runner on her high school team, and she went to college on a full scholarship. Her college coach told her she needed to drop a few pounds to be a better runner. She started a very restrictive diet, and a teammate showed her how to throw up food after a heavy meal. During her first year she developed two stress fractures in her leg that ended her track season. She was depressed that she couldn't work out and was terrified of gaining weight. She continued to diet, lost 25 pounds by her sophomore year in college, and was hospitalized with a serious case of bulimia.

Two women, both committed to being active and athletic, but two different outcomes. Why is it that today more than ever some women are "too fit to quit" while others become "too thin to win"?

Eating disorders, which might seem to be incompatible with being fit and athletic, are well known in the general population, but they have only recently been recognized in physically active women and female athletes. These disorders rob the body and mind of the energy necessary for peak performance. Active women often hide these disorders from their friends, families, and teammates.

Alarmed by the serious nature of eating disorders, members of the Women's Task Force of the American College of Sports Medicine (ACSM) called a consensus conference in 1992. Sports medicine experts, athletes, coaches, and administrators defined a new syndrome—the female athlete triad—that was causing serious problems in active women. The triad is composed of the interrelated problems of disordered eating, amenorrhea (absence of menstrual periods) and osteoporosis (thin bones).

During the conference, compelling testimony was presented about the tragic consequences of the triad, which include declining athletic performance, stress fractures, other physical and psychological problems, and even death. Because the syndrome was first identified in young female athletes, it was named the female athlete triad. But these disorders can affect women of a wide range of activity levels—not just competitive athletes. Exercising or participating in sports does not cause the triad disorders. Rather, the underlying cause of the disorders is the drive of girls and women to be unrealistically thin, often in a misguided attempt to improve their athletic performances. As a means to achieve this unrealistic thinness, many of these women turn to dieting, which in turn often spirals into disordered eating practices.

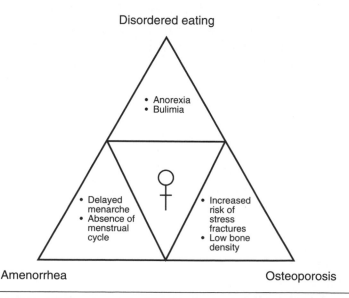

The female athlete triad is composed of three interrelated disorders—disordered eating, amenorrhea, and osteoporosis.

If a woman frequently uses disordered eating practices, she is in a state of energy drain that can lead to amenorrhea, the absence of regular menstrual cycles. Before the female athlete triad was defined, amenorrhea was mistakenly viewed as a hallmark of successful athletic training. We now know that amenorrhea is a serious sign of underlying medical problems or overtraining (see chapter 5). When a woman is amenorrheic, she lacks the hormones necessary to build bone, something the body normally does from birth to age 30. The result is a lack of healthy bone formation and irreversible bone loss, which leads to osteoporosis—old bones in young women—described in chapter 6. Women reach peak bone mass when they are between 18 and 30 years old, the same age range in which the triad is most often diagnosed.

Unlike the times in which many of us grew up, sport is now something girls and women can enjoy and compete in not only for the health benefits but also for the fun of participating, competing, and striving to push themselves to the limit. Women who are athletic are no longer viewed as abnormal. A physically active lifestyle is encouraged at all ages and for people of all abilities and interests. In this new era, in which a greater variety of sports are open to girls and women, more opportunities for college scholarships and professional sport careers are available to them. No matter what her goal is, the image of a successful woman is that she is physically active, fit, healthy, and enthused about life.

> *Fit means being physically and mentally alert and full of energy. Someone who tries her best at sports and academics is fit.*
>
> Jenny Thompson, Olympic swimmer (*Jump* magazine, April 1998)

Being fit means different things to different people. What does it mean to you to be too fit to quit? The result of being physically fit is a sense of well being and enough energy and enthusiasm to take on the challenges of life and to finish them. Our mental and physical health is enhanced by exercise. Once we used our bodies to survive; now, in a largely sedentary culture, we need physical activity even more in order to stay healthy and to avoid the medical problems that come with inactivity. In this book we emphasize being fit so that you can achieve your best—physically, emotionally, and mentally. You will learn techniques that give you higher levels of energy and enthusiasm so that you will never quit being physically active.

Being fit is exercising for your own peace of mind and being comfortable with your body. There are many different theories about how and why to exercise. But for each individual it comes down to just feeling good about yourself.

Gillian Boxx, Olympic softball player (*Jump* magazine, April 1998)

This book provides active women with practical information about being fit, developing a positive self image in today's weight-obsessed culture, and avoiding the problems of the female athlete triad. It is written for girls and women of all ages and for people who coach, parent, or advise women so that the lessons learned about the female athlete triad can be more widely disseminated and applied. We outline ways that you or someone you know can get help, and we discuss how to deal with friends, family, teammates, and coaches (chapter 7). We also provide suggestions about what can be done to prevent these serious conditions (chapter 8).

We have seen hundreds of women suffering from the triad disorders and have heard them tell the compelling stories presented on these pages. All the people in the case studies are composites drawn from women Dr. Otis has known and patients she has worked with in more than 15 years of clinical practice. As you read, you may realize that their stories remind you of women and girls you have known, perhaps even yourself.

I feel bad for kids who don't play a sport because it would totally change how they live their lives. Being fit makes you much more energized. It's not just about looking in the mirror. It's knowing that you can do things. It's feeling good about your body.

Laura Marcove, 16, high school golf, tennis, and track athlete, Riverdale, New York (*Jump* magazine, April 1998)

After the Triad Consensus Conference in 1992, we resolved to do whatever we could to recognize, treat, and prevent the triad disorders. We wrote this book in order to inform as many people as possible, and would like to hear your ideas, questions, and concerns (You can write us through our Web site, **www.sportsdoctor.com**.) We write with great love and concern for girls and women of all ages; we want to help them be the best that they can be.

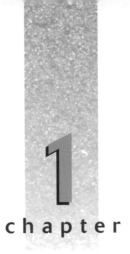

chapter

Why the Triad Now?
Developing a
Positive Body Image

There is a hidden epidemic among athletic women today. It is silently affecting their health and performance now, and it could erupt like a time bomb in the future. The female athlete triad, a syndrome comprising disordered eating, amenorrhea (missing monthly menstrual periods), and osteoporosis (thinning bones), is a serious health threat that can decimate the lives of the best and brightest women.

Do you think you are too heavy for your sport? For your age? For your best performance? Do you believe if you lost another five pounds you would be faster? Stronger? Happier? If so, then the seeds of the female athlete triad have been planted in you.

Do you closely monitor and restrict the calories you eat? Have you ever had a stress fracture? Have you missed your period for more than three months in a row? Do you occasionally vomit after you eat too much, to get rid of the calories? If you answered yes to any of these questions, then you are showing the first symptoms of the triad disorders, and you may not be as fit as you can be.

Has your mother or grandmother ever broken a hip? Is she hunched over with the painful spine fractures of osteoporosis? If so, you may be looking at your own future harvest if you suffer from the triad. Thankfully, it is a future that you can avoid.

Being an active, athletic, and healthy woman is not just about being thin or hitting the right number when you step on a scale. It's about being strong and happy, doing your body right, and celebrating the wonders of life. It means understanding yourself and loving yourself.

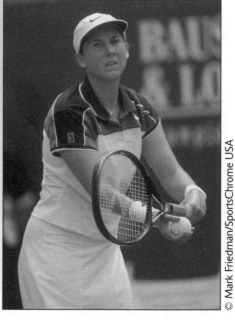

There's such a fixation with weight. It's important to be healthy, but [you] shouldn't have this fixation. It's too much pressure on women and girls. When you are young, you want to make everybody happy and you take everything personally. You want to live up to everybody's expectations. We assume that if you look thin and you look good, you must be a great person and we all love you.

Monica Seles, professional tennis player, who has close friends who have had eating disorders (*Tennis* magazine, April 1998)

© Mark Friedman/SportsChrome USA

If you are exercising intensely, not getting your periods, and obsessing about your weight, you may be hurting your performance and body more than you realize. Many competitive athletes think that losing their periods and watching precisely what they eat is part of achieving maximum fitness. Many women mistakenly equate thinness with fitness and have a distorted body image. These errors can lead to serious health and performance problems.

The female athlete triad is a relatively new syndrome; it was not recognized or described until the early 1990s. It is a syndrome born of our modern society and of Western culture's emphasis on being thin in order to be attractive and successful. It is important to know that disordered eating, amenorrhea, and loss of bone density are not caused by exercise or participation in sport or training.

The activities that lead to the triad are not the actions of a fit, high-performance woman but of one who needs professional help, because she is on a road that leads to the breakdown of her body. In this chapter we discuss the factors that affect body image in women and common ways to assess body image. Then we address some methods for improving your body image through wiser weight determinations, understanding your body type, and activities to help you reevaluate your body.

Although the disorders of the female athlete triad are serious, they are also preventable. By understanding the multiple factors leading to the triad, you, your family, your coaches, and your friends can act to resist these forces and keep from falling into the triad trap. Chapter 8 presents specific preventive strategies in detail, but first you need to understand and recognize these problems.

You can start by figuring out what being fit means to you. Is it a certain body appearance or an ability to do something? Is it an attitude or a lifestyle?

Leah was the number-one runner on her high school team. She had her pick of college scholarships and chose a PAC-Ten school with an excellent running program. However, she was only an average runner in college. Her coach told her she could be faster if she dropped a few pounds. She lost 15 pounds by fasting and running or working out twice a day her freshman year. Her cross country times improved that season, and she continued to lose weight. She then missed the whole spring season because of two stress fractures in her leg. Leah struggled to continue to keep the weight off despite her stress fractures. She restricted her diet even more because she couldn't run, and she spent twice the time in the pool or on the stationary bike instead. During her sophomore year she continued to diet, losing another 10 pounds. She was back to running, but she was not running her best times, probably because of low energy and muscle loss resulting from her restrictive dieting. She and a teammate began throwing up after eating anything they considered forbidden. She was 5'4" tall and weighed 84 pounds when she was hospitalized with bulimia over winter break during her sophomore year. We will learn more about Leah in chapter 6.

I consider a person fit if she not only feels good on the outside, but feels good on the inside. She must have good muscle tone, flexibility, and stamina. A girl doesn't have to be skinny; instead, she should have a good exercise regimen.

Dominique Dawes, Olympic gymnast (*Jump* magazine, April 1998)

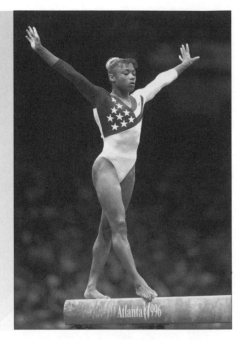

Have you ever known or heard about someone like Leah? Why is it that some athletic women turn to drastic dieting in a mistaken attempt to lose weight or perform better while others, like Olympic gymnast Dominique Dawes, keep their competitive sport and exercise in balance and stay healthy during the most strenuous competitions? Why do some women develop the interrelated problems of disordered eating, amenorrhea, and loss of bone density—known collectively as the female athlete triad—and become too thin to win?

YOUR BODY IMAGE AND THE TRIAD

The combination of disordered eating, amenorrhea, and loss of bone density was first identified in female athletes in 1992. Although these individual problems had been seen in elite women athletes for many years, it was not until then that the links between the three disorders were made. Yet the triad certainly can and does occur in women who may not consider themselves athletes but who lead physically active lives.

Think for a moment of what you feel is your idea of the right look for success as a woman and as an athlete. How tall would you be, what type of hips and thighs would you have, and what would you weigh? Is your image one of a fit, strong woman or a thin woman?

How is it different from the way you perceive yourself to look now? When asked, many men and women say that they see the ideal woman as taller and thinner than the average woman, with skinnier thighs and narrower hips. These images and the pressure to conform to them can be subtle or overt, and they clearly take hold early in a girl's life. Do you remember when you and your friends first started dieting to lose weight, and why?

We are all influenced by the cultural standards and values of the time in which we live. Think for a minute about what values are important to you. Jot down the four or five things you value the most in life.

Now write down what you value in yourself and in your friends. Many people write that their values are aspects of their personality such as loyalty, honesty, health, and the ability to care for others. But don't be surprised at how much importance you and others actually place on appearance. It is a fact of modern life; we learn that looking a certain way is desirable and we feel that our happiness is closely tied to our appearance. We know what one of the pressures underlying the development of the triad involves. It's all around us—the pressure to be thin.

Cultural Pressure: "You Can Never Be Too Thin"

Underlying the triad disorders is the pressure our culture places on women to be thin in order to be perceived as (and to feel) attractive and successful. This very real pressure can affect women of all ages, and the damage it does can last a lifetime. Even girls as young as five or six years old have been known to start dieting and to be overly concerned about their body image.

Why do we want what we don't have? Many girls and boys who are extremely thin want to gain weight and have muscles. Many girls and women with small breasts would gladly change places with their big-busted friends. Some large-breasted women wear bandage-like bras or have breast reduction surgery to be more like their smaller-breasted friends. In addition to our tendency to want what we don't have, media and advertisements inundate us with images of models who all look very similar: tall and thin, with almost no hips or thighs. As a result, in developed societies, most of us develop an unconscious drive toward the image the advertisers are selling us.

Wasn't it the Rolling Stones who said, "You can't always get what you want"? The desire for something you don't have often fuels your ambition and drive and may be what motivates you to become a "lean, mean, fighting machine." For many of us, it makes us get up each morning and work hard to achieve our dreams. It also sets up expectations and standards that are difficult to meet. Only a few people can afford to shop on Rodeo Drive in Beverly Hills or live in

Ralph Lauren country with Tommy Hilfiger, but we're bombarded with the messages that we will be happier if we buy these fashions and fit into a size-four dress.

This societal or cultural pressure to be thin leads many girls and women to unsuccessful dieting practices and quick fixes like fasting, purging, or taking diuretics and laxatives. Ultimately, confusion and myths about "normal" body weight, size, and shape often contribute to the development of disordered eating practices. These disorders can begin with what seems like innocent and perhaps harmless dieting to lose some extra pounds but they in fact trap women into a problem that can rarely be solved without professional help. They cause an energy deficit that leads to the other medical disorders of amenorrhea (lack of monthly menstrual cycles) and osteoporosis (thin bones).

Athletic Pressure: Does Thin Mean Fit?

As women have gained greater opportunities to be physically active and athletic, the larger, stronger, active woman's body has not become the ideal. Why not? Is that a threatening image? It seems strange that the stronger and more physically fit women have become, the more the waif look has become the image of attractiveness.

> *I don't think being thin or bony is attractive. I hate the way Kate Moss and the other girls who model look. I can't imagine them playing any sport, or even having fun. When I look at myself I can tell I'm athletic. I'm happy with my body. I eat whatever I want.*
>
> Janice, 19-year-old field hockey player

Understanding Body Composition

It is not news that although the female body is designed for making babies and for doing lots of other productive activities, that's not the image gracing the cover of Cosmopolitan. Before puberty, boys and girls are pretty much equal in body type, body composition, and even athletic performance. Then comes puberty. Hormones are activated, causing many changes in the body. This riot of estrogen and progesterone starts for girls about two years before boys are attacked by their own special hormone—testosterone. Testosterone makes guys grow taller, aquire more muscle mass, develop bigger and stronger bones and hearts, and produce more red blood cells. All these changes make guys the stronger sex of the human species.

For women, estrogen and progesterone increase breast size, hip girth, and percentage of body fat.

One result of the hormones of puberty is a significant difference between the body compositions of men and women. What do you think is a normal body fat percentage for a woman?

The body composition differences between men and women after puberty are shown in figure 1.1. Note that males have 40 to 55 percent muscle mass and 14 to 20 percent body fat. Women have less muscle mass—35 to 50 percent—and more body fat.

Average women in the United States have 18 to 35 percent body fat. Although women who are physically active may have somewhat lower body fat percentages than the average, depending on their type of training and their genetically determined set point, typically, if a woman's body fat percentage is below 16, she is considered too thin for good health. And in most cases, she is also too thin to win.

Does it surprise you that a healthy woman's body fat percentage is this high? Is your understanding of normal body fat in line with the facts? If not, where did your idea of a normal or desired body fat

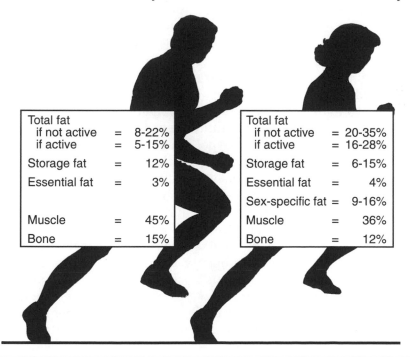

Figure 1.1 Different body compositions of average men and women. Notice that women's higher body fat levels (over men's) are due to a necessary amount of sex-specific fat stores.

percentage come from? A scientific article, a discussion with a physician or nutritionist, or a conversation with a friend? Please understand that it is normal for women to have more body fat than our society deems appropriate. There is a critical amount of body fat that is necessary to be healthy. Contrary to our notions that all fat is bad, fat plays an important and specific role in the health of our bodies and minds.

Body fat comes in three different types: storage, essential, and (for women) sex-specific. Storage fat is the type of fat that is gained or lost the most. It is the type that surrounds and cushions our organs and is deposited under the skin. Our bodies have the ability to put in deposits and make withdrawals from the storage fat as an energy reserve. About 6 to 15 percent of a woman's body is made up of storage fat. About 8 to 12 percent of a man's body is storage fat. Both men and women have about 3 to 4 percent essential fat. This fat is stored in the bone marrow, heart, liver, and central nervous system. This fat is absolutely necessary for the functioning of these organs and for maintenance of the immune system.

The major difference between body composition in men and women is that women have an additional component known as sex-specific fat—approximately 9 to 16 percent of their total body weight. It is stored principally in the hips, thighs, pelvis, and breasts and is needed for normal reproductive functions, including regular menstrual periods, pregnancy, and lactation. It is difficult to decrease this component of body fat even with dieting. There are genetic differences in the amount and the location of this component of body fat. However, a woman may experience difficulty with her reproductive functions if she loses too much of her sex-specific body fat.

In the 1950s, a few people starting pinching other people and writing down numbers. The pinchers were scientists studying body composition. They knew that most of the body (70 percent, in fact) was water, but what about the rest? They found that people are made of fat, bone, muscle, and finally, the remainders—guts, gristle, and whatever else you can imagine but don't want to think about. They devised ways to measure different body components, but they had a hard time getting reasonably accurate measurements on live people. They ended up with measurement techniques that were only estimates of body fat.

Body fat hides in many places in the body, not just under the skin. By doing skinfold measurements, scientists were not really getting the whole picture; they were only assessing the 70 to 80 percent of fat that is stored under the skin. This type of indirect measurement is based on many assumptions about the body and leaves room for a wide range of error. Moreover, the estimates require various equations that are specific for different types of people and for race, gender, and activity levels. Scientists found that to be most accurate, the measurements must be taken very precisely with standardized machines and by people who are experienced in using these machines.

Given all the estimates and guesswork inherent in this type of measurement, the range of error for body fat determinations is anywhere from 3.5 to 12 percent. In the best hands, the error range is plus or minus 3.9 percent when testing is done on young, physically active women. This means if you have 17 percent body fat (which could only be accurately determined by dissecting your body if you died on the day of the test), you could be told that you have anywhere from 13 to 21 percent body fat. In reality, given this true range of error, body fat percentage should always be reported as a range rather than as one figure!

The overemphasis placed on body composition testing is another factor that has led some people to develop disordered eating patterns. Women whose body fat percentage is reported as higher than they desire can be panicked into inappropriate dieting or disordered eating. Only recently has body composition testing entered the sport science and medicine fields. However, before we knew how to pinch a skin fold or weigh someone under water, bright, intelligent people were coaching athletic girls and women to compete successfully. Women were even winning gold medals and setting personal bests.

Better Body Composition Testing

There is a lot of confusion about body composition testing. Some coaches and trainers would have you believe that your percentage of body fat determines your fitness, performance, success, motivation, desire, and adherence to a training regimen. Nothing could be further from the truth. You just can't put all your eggs in one basket like this.

Rather, it is important to make sure that you establish positive, healthful goals for the assessment before you submit to any body composition testing. One goal might be to determine your muscle to fat ratio. Sometimes women are told they are too heavy, but body composition testing indicates that their body fat percentages are low and their muscle mass is high. These women would find it extremely difficult (and detrimental to their athletic performance) to lose weight. Another goal might be to use the assessment as a way of monitoring body composition changes throughout a training season.

Determining the ideal body weight and body composition for success in sport is not a realistic goal. It is illogical and inaccurate to think that there is one ideal body fat percentage for a given sport. If any measurement is done, it should be to determine the amount and quality of muscle rather than body fat. A coach or athlete who is effectively attempting to achieve an optimum body composition for a sport is really trying to change body composition so that the percentage of lean tissue (muscle) is optimal. Assessments should therefore emphasize lean body (muscle) composition.

Can You Enhance Performance By Losing Weight or Body Fat?

You must take several factors into account before assuming that athletic performance will be enhanced by weight loss. The relationship between body composition and performance is more complex than one measurement can determine. Factors you should consider include the following:

◆ What is your sport and what are its components for success? If it requires muscular power and strength, then loss of muscle will be detrimental.

◆ The thinner you are, the lower the chances are that your performance will benefit from weight loss. You will increase the risk of becoming too thin and this will detrimentally affect your performance.

◆ Rapid weight loss, or weight loss during the competitive season, can impair rather than enhance your performance, particularly if you lose lean body mass (muscle).

◆ Your method of attempted weight loss can impair performance by resulting in dehydration, loss of muscle, and loss of fuel for sport.

◆ The higher the level of performance you have achieved before losing weight, the lower the potential performance improvement from that weight loss.

◆ If a medical professional says weight loss is indicated for you, it must take place gradually, at no more than one-half to one pound per week and under the supervision of a nutritionist or other medical personnel. At this rate, muscle is preserved. The best time for you to lose weight is during the off-season.

Can body composition measurement predict athletic success? The answer is no. No one measurement can tell you if you are fit or fat. It cannot tell if you have been training hard, eating right, and following the dictums of a good, informed coach. As previously noted, body composition measurements, at their best, can only tell you what range of body fat percentages you fall into, because these measurements have large margins of error. More mistakes have been made and more athletic careers destroyed by over-reliance on body composition measurement than for almost any other reason.

Interpreting Test Results

For purposes of comparison, we've detailed the accuracy of several of the different types of body composition measurements (table 1.1). The gold standard has been underwater weighing—a technique that is not easily available—but even that technique has an error range of plus or minus 3.5 percent. Many new techniques purporting to be highly accurate have been developed, marketed, and (mis)used. If you decide to have a body composition measurement done, or if you base any decisions about diet or weight goals on such a measurement, carefully review the technique used and the experience of the measurer, and have several repeat measurements done to ensure accuracy. However, unless you have clearly stated goals, we do not recommend doing these measurements because of their inaccuracy and the potential for their results to be misinterpreted.

Although tables of ideal ranges of body composition for athletes in various sports are published, these tables were generated without knowing the athletes' genetic makeups, body types, diet patterns, or training regimens, or the margin of error of the measurement techniques used. Jack Wilmore, PhD, an exercise scientist and author of some early tables illustrating body fat percentages in athletes, has since made the following statement:

> *Published standards of mean values for relative body fat for small numbers of athletes are arbitrary. They do not recognize measurement error, the wide variation in body fat percentage associated with successful performance, and the genetic variation within a given somatotype. If standards must be established, a range of values that recognize both individual variability and methodological error should be set. The upper limit of the range should be justified for the individual and attainable with the least risk of precipitating disordered eating. The lower limit of the range should represent the lowest value achieved by elite performers who are healthy and exhibit no signs or symptoms of disordered eating* (Wilmore in Otis et al., 1997).

Table 1.1					
Ratings of the Validity and Objectivity of Body Composition Methods					
Method	**Precise**	**Objective**	**Accurate**	**Valid equations**	**Overall**
Body mass index	1	1	4,5	4,5	4
Near-infrared interactance	1	1,2	4	4	3.5
Skinfolds	2	2,3	2,3	2,3	2.5
Bioelectric impedance	2	2	2,3	2,3	2.5
Circumferences	2	2	2,3	2,4	3.0

1=Excellent, 2=Very good, 3=Good, 4=Fair, 5=Unacceptable

Precise refers to the repeatability of the method in the hands of the same investigator over several trials. **Objective** refers to the comparability of the method between investigatiors. **Accurate** refers to the criterion-related validity or the comparability of a method with an accepted reference method or criterion method (e.g., underwater weighting). **Valid equations** means that equations that have been published on a given population using a given method have been cross-validated on other samples of the same population and found effective.

Reprinted, by permission, from T. Lohmann, L. Houtkooper, and S.B. Going, 1997, "Body fat measurement goes high-tech," *ACSM's Health and Fitness Journal* 1(1):30-34.

Many people have been misled in their pursuit of health, happiness, and the ideal body by having a body composition measurement done. One young gymnast I cared for had a body fat measurement done at her local health club. The technique was a bioelectrical impedance study, and it involved the use of a new piece of equipment just purchased by the club. Club staff members were offering free measurements while they learned to use the machinery. This gymnast had trained hard and had dieted all summer. By her scale she had lost two pounds. She felt good about the progress she had made over the summer, because she had put some new elements into her tumbling routine and her uniform was fitting well.

When she went for the body composition testing at her local gym, she was unaware that the machine was new and was not standardized. In fact, it did not have standards of comparison for young, thin girls. She was told her body fat was 23 percent, high for her expectations as a competitive athlete. She immediately went on a strict starvation program and ultimately lost a lot of her lean muscle. She admitted that she was tired and depressed, and she felt that all her good workouts had been for nothing—based solely on this one measurement. She went back to be measured again two weeks later, and she was told that her body fat had increased to 26 percent. She was in despair.

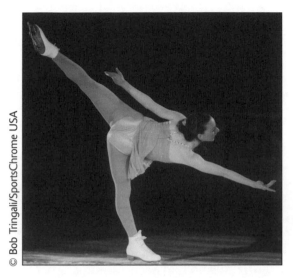

© Bob Tringali/SportsChrome USA

Body composition measurements are less reliable in assessing your fitness than other measures of sports-specific skills and attributes.

In spite of her hard training, lean body, and the fact that she was feeling good, the gymnast chose to believe this magical machine. She was terror stricken and believed she was too fat to compete in gymnastics. She returned to school two weeks later, anxious, dieting, and worried. During her physical for the team, she revealed what had happened over the summer and how desperate she was to lose all the body fat she had mysteriously "gained." In fact, she had not gained any body fat. Rather, she had been the victim of a new machine and a formula that was in error for her body type.

We did another measurement on the gymnast, the sum of her skinfold thickness. This number is not converted into body fat percentage and is more emotionally neutral. We had used this measurement in previous years, and we found that it was essentially the same as the prior year. I told her about the high error range in the impedance study, and we called her club to ask what machine they were using. We found out that the machine used one formula for all people. It was a formula for middle-aged people, and it was not standardized for her. Relieved, she disregarded that measurement and began concentrating on continuing her healthy diet and training.

We have challenged the misuse of body composition measurements with coaches, trainers, parents, athletes, and strength and conditioning coaches time and time again. They often tell us they need to have these measurements to see if the athlete is training correctly. It is more likely that they would be able to tell if an athlete is training right by her performance, her willingness to work out, her energy level, how she moves, and by measurements of specific attributes relevant to the given sport, such as speed, strength, and endurance.

◤The Basketball Team

Concerned about having a fit, competitive team, one college basketball coach required that all her players have a body fat percentage of 17 percent or less before they were given their uniforms. Of course, without their uniforms they could not play! The team members knew of the requirement, but they had no way of knowing their body compositions.

How did the coach pick this number? She read a table of ideal body composition measurements indicating that women basketball players should have body fat percentages between 15 and 21 percent. (I never received a satisfactory explanation as to why she picked 17 percent.) The team members were very anxious about having this measurement done. Many of them had not eaten the day before M (measurement) day and had been "dieting" (that is, starving themselves) for weeks in order to pass the test. However, they stuffed themselves the night before the test, when their willpower was finally overwhelmed by hunger.

They all felt nervous about M day, and some of them unconsciously overate for that reason. Do any of these behaviors sound familiar to you? Not surprisingly, M day was a disaster. Most of the shorter players with stockier builds "flunked" the test. The players who were naturally tall, thin, and lean did okay. The ones who flunked were humiliated, had to do extra running drills, and were not given their uniforms.

When the medical staff heard about this strange requirement (at least it was strange to us and should be to you, now that you know the realities of body composition measurement), we were able to convince the athletic administrators to drop it and let the team get their uniforms and start practice. Several girls later told me that they developed serious problems about eating just from their experience with this one requirement.

Understanding Body Types

Like it or not, in addition to inheriting your body composition tendencies, to a degree you inherit a certain body type (see pages 18 to 20 for a discussion of various body types) just as you inherit a certain height and eye color. Blame your parents and their genes if you can't fit into your jeans! Human nature being what it is, most of us dislike what we have and want something else.

Think about this for yourself and some of your friends. What is it that you want but can't have? Is it blue eyes if yours are hazel? What about your friends? The short ones may want to be taller, whereas the tall ones might give anything to be shorter. This desire to be something we are not is common and is almost a normal part of life. It is what keeps beauty salons in business and makes plastic surgeons the best-paid doctors around. The desire and the efforts to be thin are what lead to the serious disorders of the female athlete triad.

Expectations of how we should look are clearly influenced by society and not by the body type we inherit. Standards of beauty change over the years. And, paradoxically, the preferred body type is often one that is rare, difficult to attain, and not achievable by many people in society or in athletics.

Come with us on a trip back in time. Think of the desired body type for women in prehistoric times. They were tough times, when fast food meant running down a rabbit, then skinning and grilling it. In these tough times, a well-rounded, fertile, even plump woman was the ideal. Not too many women could achieve that look, considering McDonald's was thousands of years in the future. In fact, it was almost impossible to get fat with all the hunting, gathering, and famine that was the norm for life in 3000 BC.

The fat woman was the fertile woman, and thus the ideal woman in that society; she was the cover woman of the Stone Age Vogue. She had enough body fat to survive two years of drought, enough fat to get pregnant and nurse a child. Any man could see how valuable she was to his plans for establishing a dynasty or surviving the next famine. And this woman was a rare woman. Not many women could look like her, unless they overate or genetically inherited a body type that stored fat easily. Over the years, more women inherited this body type, because it allowed them to survive the times of famine. They passed along this successful body type to their descendants. We recognize women with this body type today. They have inherited a beautiful body type that is idealized in many societies where fertility and survival are valued. For example, some Samoan, Fijian, Eskimo, and Pima Indian women have this body type, because it has helped them survive the rigors of their lives.

Do you have any friends or family members who have this body type? If so, see the beauty in it and the success it represents. Most of the members of the human species have either been at or are on the brink of starvation. Today, there are vast areas of the world where people are starving or facing drought because of political conflict or environmental changes. People with robust, strong, healthy bodies will be more likely to survive.

> **"Y**ou've gained weight," used to be a compliment in the Fiji culture, where a full-figured, robust body was a sign of health and wealth. However, a 1999 Harvard Medical School study of women in Fiji reported an increase of disordered eating practices after exposure to Western television shows. Among high school girls, disordered eating (vomiting) increased from 3 to 15 percent from 1995 to 1998. The percentage of women who tested high for eating disorder risk more than doubled during this time period. These changes in behavior came three years after Fijians' only television channel started broadcasting shows like "Melrose Place," "Beverly Hills 90210," and "Xena, Warrior Princess." One girl said that her friends "changed their mood, their hairstyles, so that they can be more like those characters. So in order to be like them, I have to work on myself, exercising, and my eating habits should change."
>
> Reported in *The New York Times*, May 20, 1999.

In today's Western culture, the very body type that ensured the survival of the human race is not popular. What image do you have

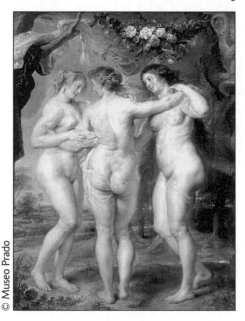

© Museo Prado

of women who are heavy? Some people judge heavy women by their appearance and categorize them as lazy, unwilling to exercise, or weak-willed. Recently, Jay Leno did a comedy skit on his TV show. He took a copy of the painting "Three Graces" by Rubens and showed it to people in the street (see figure 1.2). His question to them was, "Could these women get a date in Los Angeles today?" The response was a resounding and unanimous, "No!" Although Leno milked this for laughs, it was a very telling commentary on the perception of beauty in women today.

Figure 1.2   Jay Leno asked of Peter Paul Rubens's "Three Graces," "Could these women get a date in Los Angeles today?" The audience responded, "No!"

Cultural values for beauty change with the times. As we've already noted, the unusual woman, the one whose body type is difficult to achieve, has often been idolized. Women have often gone to extremes to achieve the ideal body type for their time. Think of Scarlet O'Hara in *Gone With the Wind*. She had her maids mercilessly cinch her waist in tight corsets. How did she ride horses or dance, much less even breathe? In the 1920s a tomboyish Flapper was the ideal, and large-breasted women were "out of style." A well-rounded Marilyn Monroe with natural hips, thighs, and even a small stomach bulge became an icon of the ideal in the 1950s and 1960s. And what about Twiggy hitting in the late sixties? Styles come and go, yet all women are affected in some way by the style of their times. How does the current image of beauty affect you? What does it make you think about your body? What do you think is the ideal body type and look? Take a minute and write down what kind of body you think is beautiful. Why do you think it is beautiful?

> *The* he average female fashion model is considerably different from the average American woman. The average model is 5'9" tall and weighs 110 pounds. The average woman is 5'4" and weighs 140 pounds.
>
> Source: *ETR Associates Handbook*

Most girls and women find they do not measure up to what they see as the ideal. The desirable female body shape in our culture is usually not attainable by a normal woman, nor is it a shape that is easily or healthily achieved. We have many images of the women who represent the cultural ideal available to us on TV, in magazines, on the Internet, and in movies. It is important to realize, when looking at photos of these women, that they have spent hours being worked on by professional make-up artists and stylists to achieve their "naturally thin" look. Also, the photographs are taken at angles that unnaturally elongate the models' legs, and then are sometimes computer-enhanced to make the women appear thinner and younger.

Some of the women who appear in magazines or on TV have had surgery to look the way they do. Some have developed eating disorders and the female athlete triad and are seriously ill. They are not hard to spot once you know what to look for. As an exercise in awareness, pick up any modern women's magazine and flip through the pages. Notice how the images are distorted to make the women appear a certain way. Are these natural ways of standing or moving? Do they look like anyone you see in real life? Notice which models are extremely thin and gaunt looking. They may be suffering from anorexia, a very severe eating disorder that has a 15 percent death rate. Begin to reject these images as ideal or even as normal and healthy. This can be a very liberating exercise. Try to find images of women who look real, who look healthy and physically fit, and use them as your role models.

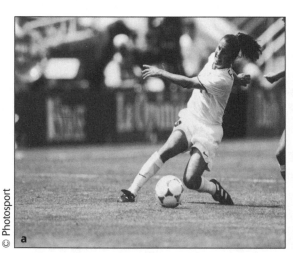
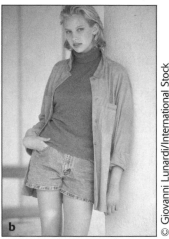

It's not difficult to find images of healthy, active women to embrace as role models (a) instead of the more static, often distorted, fashion model shots (b) often seen in magazines.

What Is Your Body Type?

In addition to the differences in body composition between boys and girls, we also inherit a certain body type. These body types are recognizable from afar, usually just by looking at someone's outline.

Knowing and accepting your body type can help you understand how to be fit, healthy, and happy. After all, we know that body type is inherited and resists any change, whether through dieting or overeating. But many people—athletes, coaches, and parents alike—do not recognize body types and do not understand the implications of body type on sport selection, weight gain and loss, and body composition.

A college softball player who played catcher and center field was repeatedly told by her coach that she would be faster if she would just lose a few pounds. Many athletic women have heard those words at one time or another. If you hear them yourself, do not listen! Speed has a great deal to do with muscle type and power, and type of training, not just how much you weigh. If you need to get faster, train specifically for speed. Do not diet.

This player attended a college that required body composition testing (this was back in the Dark Ages of women's sports, before athletic departments knew better). Her body fat percentage came out at 15 percent, a very low number considering that with the error range it might have been anywhere from 11 to 19 percent. Her coach was incredulous, and the athlete was ecstatic. The trainer repeated the test three times, using the skinfold technique. And the repeat figures again were between 15 and 17 percent. This girl has a strong, healthy body with a lot of muscle and not very much fat. Had she been pressured to diet and lose more weight, she would have lost muscle. And the result? You guessed it. Losing lean muscle mass would have made her slower, weaker, more easily fatigued, and so forth. So, sometimes a body composition measurement can help if there is a dispute about whether a person needs to lose weight, but it's still not holy scripture. As we have discussed, determinations about weight goals are best made by medical staff.

There are three main body types, and then there are blends of those types. The three main types are the ectomorph, mesomorph, and endomorph (figure 1.3). Ectomorphs are tall and thin and have long arms and legs. These people have difficulty gaining weight and muscle. They have the body type you tend to see in ballet dancers, models, high jumpers, and long-distance runners. Mesomorphs are muscular, shorter, and have stocky arms and legs. These people are strong and tend to gain muscle mass when they do strength training. They may find it difficult to lose weight, but they excel in power sports like soccer, softball, and sprinting events in track and field. Endomorphs are shaped like apples or pears and carry more body fat. Sports they excel at are distance swimming, field events, and weight lifting. In between the general types are blends of types. Many of us are blends; for example, Natalie, the basketball player just quoted, is a blend of an ectomorph and a mesomorph type. Women who excel in sports that emphasize power are often mesomorphs or blends of mesomorphs and ectomorphs. However, body type doesn't necessarily determine your success or failure in any given sport, nor should it preclude you from participating in a sport you like. A classic example is Joan Benoit Samuelson, winner of the first women's Olympic marathon. Even with her mesomorphic body type, she succeeded in a sport usually dominated by ectomorphs.

Each body type has advantages over others for certain activities, but a person with any body type can be physically fit. Whatever body type you have can usually be seen in your family. You may take after your father's (mesomorphic) side of the family, and your sister may look more like your mother's (ectomorphic) side. If you choose a certain sport and get really interested in it, you will find that some body types are preferred for different sports. Think how important being an ectomorph is for success in ballet. A young girl who has all the desire and drive in the world to be a great ballerina

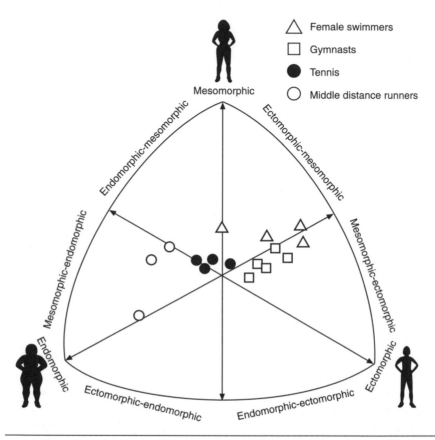

Figure 1.3 The unique advantages of a particular body type can influence the degree of success possible in a given sport.

Reprinted, by permission, from J.A. Wessel, 1972, *Movement Fundamentals: Figure, Form, Fun,* 3rd ed. (Englewood Cliffs, NJ: Prentice Hall), 223.

might have a mesomorphic body. She might find that her ectomorphic classmates are chosen for the lead roles even though she may technically be the better dancer.

Christine loved running because of the sense of freedom and control it gave her. She was determined to be a great runner, and she read all she could about successful women runners. She ran cross country in high school and wanted to become a marathon runner. She had posters and pictures of some of the great runners of the past and present, like Grete Waitz, Ingrid Kristiansen, and Anne Marie Lauck. They all seemed a lot thinner than she was, and they had almost no thigh fat.

Christine trained as hard as anyone on her cross country team, but she was not the number-one runner. No matter how hard she trained, she thought she could see fat in her thighs. It jiggled when she ran unless she had on really tight bike shorts. She wore those shorts most of the time, because she hated her fat thighs. One day at practice, she noticed that the number-one and number-two runners on her team were wearing really high-cut running shorts ("bun huggers"). When these runners bent over to stretch their hamstrings, she could see they had no thigh fat. Also, she could see the bones of their spines through their running tops. Christine was determined to get rid of any thigh fat and have a thin back so her skeleton would show, too. She thought that was the way to become a better runner.

She undertook a strict plan of fasting every other day and eating only nonfat foods on alternate days. She lost a pound over the next week, but she was not running faster. She did two hundred side leg lifts a day to get rid of thigh fat. She felt fat every time she looked at the posters of the great marathoners and her thin teammates. Christine was unhappy and lost her joy in running. She thought if she could only look like them, she would be a great and happy runner.

Christine didn't recognize that she was a natural mesomorph and that her ideal distance runners were natural ectomorphs. No matter how many leg lifts she did or how much weight she lost, she would never look like Grete Waitz. A wise friend who knew about different body types saw what was happening to Christine. It had happened to her, too. She was a mesomorph living in an ectomorph world. What to do about it? There is no way you can change the fact that people who have bodies naturally suited to their sports are going to be successful. They are the lucky ones, the ones the coaches pick out in the early years. But you can learn to love your own body and to maximize your potential. Christine's coach put her in with the 400-meter runners. The shorter distance was easy for her and much more suited to her strength and naturally muscular body type. She felt strong, successful, and happy in the new event. Her attitude changed, and her times improved as she developed more speed and strength for the shorter run. Once she stopped comparing herself to thinner ectomorphic runners, she relaxed her strict dieting. She felt more satisfied as her training improved.

How can you be successful, healthy, and happy in a sport or activity that you love?

1. Realize that you cannot change your body type. Learn to love and respect your body and to work with what you have.

2. Stop comparing yourself to others. This is incredibly destructive and self-defeating behavior. You can never have someone else's curly hair, long legs, or ectomorphic build.

3. Celebrate your body and the marvelous things it can do when you are fit and well nourished. Keep your body healthy and happy. Body type alone does not determine success in sport or happiness in life. Know what you like to do, what you enjoy, what interests and excites you. And go for it!

Body Types and Sports

Girls who have not gone through puberty may perform better in gymnastics than those with more "womanly" bodies. The small, compact, prepubertal body goes through space faster and can more easily do tricks that involve tumbling and somersaults. If gymnastics judges preferred a more mature body type and the artistry of a choreographed routine rather than the tricks of tiny youth, then the sport of gymnastics would again be a woman's instead of a child's sport.

These ideals are variable and change with the culture. They emphasize youth and, paradoxically, a type of body that is nearly impossible to attain unless you were born into it. There is a great deal of truth in the saying that if you were not born with it, you can't have it. If you were not born to have the ectomorph body of a model like Kate Moss (remember, blame your parents' genes for this one, not yourself), then you never will. You can drive yourself crazy trying to look like the latest gold-medal Olympic gymnast if you were born with the body of a shot putter. When women in sport are pressured by themselves or others to become a different body type or to lose unrealistic amounts of weight, they are at risk for developing the female athlete triad.

It is true that certain body types may do slightly better in some sports and activities. But being fit and healthy can come in any size and shape. We find the most female athlete triad problems in women who have the desire to achieve in certain sports (gymnastics, figure skating, long distance running) or professions (modeling or dance), but do not have the "preferred" body type for that activity. They struggle to change their bodies to fit the mold desired in this particular sport or activity, rather than enjoying the sport or activity for itself. If your body type does not fit the sport you like, you can still enjoy the sport for the fun of it. Not everyone has to be an exact body fit for sport to enjoy the thrill of victory (figure 1.4).

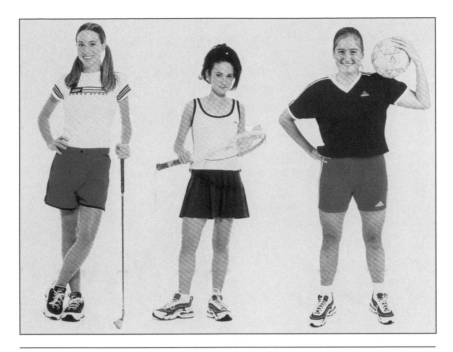

Figure 1.4 Healthy, athletic women come in all sizes and shapes.

TOWARD A HEALTHY BODY IMAGE

I never weigh myself. I threw out my scale years ago. I can tell how I feel by how my clothes fit and how much energy I have. I'm an average-size person, but well toned. I never diet. I like food too much and I like feeling good. If I gain a few pounds, I know as soon as I start working out again, I can lose that weight in a few weeks.

Carol Ann, an aerobics teacher

Reevaluating your body image means recognizing that your ideal body weight is simply the range where you feel healthy and fit, have no signs of an eating disorder to maintain that weight, and have healthy, functioning immune and reproductive systems. That's right; there is no table listing the "correct" weight that you should compare yourself to and no specific number on the scale that you should be shooting for. It is easier to aim for feeling fit, healthy, and happy. We are all so programmed to think there is a magical body weight that will make us happy that it is a real act of revolution to throw out the scale in favor of feeling well.

*E*veryone in my family is big and I like being that way. I enjoy being noticed and being stronger than most other people, even guys. I would hate to be a thin, fragile, anorectic type because I wouldn't be able to do the things I love to do. I play two sports in college and being fit is my way of life.

Natalie, a 5'11", 175-pound forward on her college basketball team.

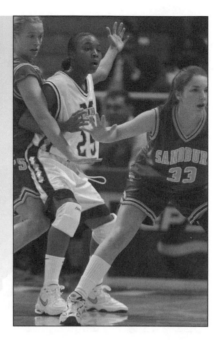

Yes, there are plenty of tables that tell you what you "should" weigh. Those that are most often referenced are ancient. The Metropolitan Life Insurance tables were first produced in the 1950s and have been reproduced as though they were some holy scripture since then. These ideal weight guides have long been proved wrong, but they are still used in many doctor's offices, in articles in women's magazines, and even in scientific documents. Each of us has our own set point for body weight (see the following section) according to our body type. Variations in body type are not taken into account by these tables. Trying to achieve a certain weight based on information in a table, particularly if the table is inaccurate, can lead you to unnecessary dieting and to disordered eating practices.

Your Set Point

Why, in spite of all the differences in food and exercise from week to week, does body weight stay the same? Researchers have found that each of us has a set point, a weight at which our body is programmed to stay. Our body resists changes in weight and stays within a few pounds of our set point, which is a weight that is healthy for us. The set point acts like a thermostat in your house that is set at a specific temperature. It is great to have a thermostat that automatically keeps the house warm in winter and cool in summer. We can change that thermostat setting to match the season.

The thermostat in the body that sets weight is not so easily changed. This "weight-o-stat" is controlled by the body's master gland, the hypothalamus. It is programmed to keep you in a certain weight range set by factors that you inherit from your parents. Your genetic inheritance includes all kinds of things, from hair color to height to your tendency to get certain diseases. You can no more change these inherited genetic traits than you can change the color of your eyes. Well, we take some of that back. People can use tinted contact lenses to "change" the color of their eyes and permanent waves to change straight hair to curly hair for a while. But basically, what you see is what you get.

Wiser Weight Determinations

The use of body composition testing out of the context of a total plan and program for monitoring health and fitness has induced so much fear, dieting, and disordered eating that it should be abolished. Athletes often develop the disorders of the female athlete triad because their coaches or others subject them to mandatory weigh-ins, inaccurate body composition tests, unrealistic weight goals, and derogatory or sarcastic comments about their weight.

In an attempt to reduce the pressure on female athletes, several college athletic programs have eliminated weigh-ins entirely and have had very successful outcomes. These include improved performance and better athlete–coach relationships. If you are stuck in a program that still does body composition testing, there are several paths you can take to make things easier on you and on your coach as well.

There are several excellent models for determining appropriate weight goals for athletes. The one that we endorse and that has stood the test of time is the program shown in figure 1.5 that was developed by the University of Texas Performance Team, which is lead by Randa Ryan, PhD.

This plan recognizes that weight is an issue for female athletes and their coaches. It recognizes that the proper procedure for dealing with weight issues is in consultation with trained sport science and medicine professionals. Ask most coaches and they will tell you they would be relieved not to have to address weight issues with their female athletes. Coaches are trained for and excel at motivating, drilling, and training athletes. When the weight issue rears its ugly head, many coaches feel that they are not prepared to deal with it. Coaches should consult with professionals who are trained to work in this area and may turn these issues completely over to nutritionists and other professionals.

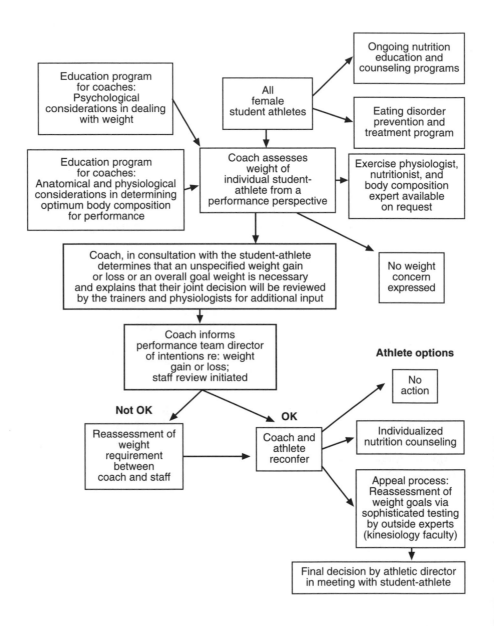

Figure 1.5 A recommended program to help coaches and student-athletes make wise weight management decisions.

Reprinted, by permission, from R. Ryan, 1992, "Management of eating problems in athletic settings." In *Eating, Body Weight and Performance in Athletes: Disorders of Modern Society*, edited by K.D. Brownell, J. Rodin, and J.H. Wilmore (Philadelphia: Lea and Febiger), 344-360.

If you are not on an athletic team, but you are physically active and feel pressured or concerned about your weight, what should you do? These are indications you should seek professional advice and you can find help within this model. Start by asking your primary care physician, a nutritionist, a nurse practitioner, or another clinician about what a reasonable weight range is for you. First, determine whether your weight concerns are realistic or not. Have your weight and eating habits monitored by professionals, and follow up frequently with visits to check your health and nutritional status. You can then reassure yourself or others who are concerned that the "weight issue" is being evaluated.

Preventing the triad begins with developing realistic weight goals and eliminating undue weight pressure from yourself, coaches, trainers, parents, and others. Trained professionals can help you establish a management plan and a weight goal. All plans should emphasize health, fitness, and balance—not just weight loss. If you gained 10 pounds the first year in college or when you started a new job, then start a sound nutrition and exercise plan. You and your professional advisors should agree on any weight plan and goal. If you disagree with their assessment, then discuss it openly with your advisors.

Effective Weight Control

If you have gained weight, you may need some nutrition education and direction in effective weight control techniques (see sidebar, page 28). A counselor can help you identify behavioral factors that lead to overeating and can teach you how to change your patterns so that you eat in response to hunger rather than as a reaction to stress or anxiety.

If you do not carefully assess your situation and set a realistic weight goal, your weight loss program will not be successful. Very few people learn how to effectively lose weight on their own, especially during a stressful time or a competitive season. Finding professionals to help you is often easier if you are an athlete in high school or college than it is if you are out of school and don't have that kind of institutional support. Find out what resources are available through your health care system or through programs like Weight Watchers. You can construct your own support team by finding the right nutritionist, exercise physiologist, primary care practitioner, and counselor. Peer and nonprofessional support groups also exist (for example, Overeaters Anonymous).

If you are like most girls and women, you have tried several practices that may not be very effective for losing weight and keeping it off. Some typical techniques and their results are listed in table 1.2 (see p 31).

Healthy Eating and Effective Weight Management

Healthy eating means fueling your body for everything it needs to do. Eating well gives you energy and helps you appreciate food as nourishment and not see it as your enemy. Effective weight management involves lifestyle changes and adjusting how you think and act around food. Successful plans are based on realistic goals, eating normal food, and incorporating regular exercise into your life.

Set Realistic Goals

* Ask yourself if you need to lose weight or if you just need to eat better for your health and sport performance?
* Work with a professional to determine a realistic weight range based on your body type, past weight history, general health, and menstrual cycle status.
* If you determine that you need to lose weight, aim for weight loss no more than 1/2 to 1 pound a week during training. Do not choose as your goal the lowest weight you have ever been (or the smallest size of clothes you ever wore).
* Weigh yourself no more than once a week, if at all.

Choose a Plan for Healthy Eating

* Work with a professional, such as a registered dietitian.
* Avoid fad diets. They do not work in the long run.
* Make a plan for your eating that meets your energy needs.
* Make shopping lists and plan ahead so you are less tempted to eat on the spur of the moment or to pick high-fat fast food.
* Have readily available low-calorie, high-nutrition snacks like fruit, veggies, and air-popped popcorn.
* If you've determined you need to lose weight, reduce your daily caloric intake by 200 to 300 calories and increase your daily exercise by 20 minutes.

Keep Moving

* Exercise four to six times a week.
* Choose a mix of aerobic activity (for 30 minutes each bout) and strength training (for 20 minutes each bout), to build muscle as well as boost your metabolic rate.

- If you are frustrated by working out a lot and not losing weight, add a longer bout of aerobic exercise at a slower pace once a week to boost your energy expenditure. Try a long hike or a bike ride of 90 minutes if you are ready for it.
- Emphasize the large muscles of the body such as the upper arms, legs, and gluteal areas.

Increase Your Metabolic Rate

- Avoid starvation, which lowers your metabolic rate.
- Eat breakfast.
- Eat small, frequent meals 4 to 6 times a day.
- If you are a chronic dieter, it may take 4 to 12 weeks to restore your metabolic rate to normal. Be patient.

Eliminate Empty Calories

- Avoid alcohol.
- Avoid high-fat snacks such as chips and dips. Fat has more than twice the calories of other foods.
- Avoid simple sugars in certain drinks (sodas, etc.) and foods. These foods are very dense in calories but low in nutrition.

Increase Your Fluid Intake

- Drink at least 8 large glasses of water a day. This will fill you up, keep you from being dehydrated, and help your athletic performance.
- Drink a large glass of water before eating or before a problem situation for overeating. This will help you to eat less.

Downsize Your Portions

- Cut in half the amount of each portion you that usually eat.
- Don't deny yourself a piece of dessert if you love it, but take a smaller portion.
- Use smaller bowls and plates at home.
- In restaurants, choose half portions or plan to take some food home.

Develop New Habits

- Don't eat in front of the TV or a book. Set a place setting and concentrate on enjoying the food rather than rushing through and possibly overeating.

(continued)

Healthy Eating (continued)

◆ Know your eating patterns from your food-mood diary. People who keep a record are more aware of their behaviors, thoughts, and feelings and of how these connect to eating.

◆ Take at least 20 minutes to eat. It takes that amount of time for your stomach to tell your brain that you are full. Take time to chew your food thoroughly, put your fork down between bites, and enjoy your food.

◆ Identify what triggers your eating and learn how to better manage your feelings. Use techniques that help you nurture and comfort yourself instead of relying on food.

Find Solutions to Problem Foods and Situations

◆ Make a list of your problem foods and contrast it with tasty substitutes.

◆ List problem situations in which you are likely to overeat or blow your plan, and come up with solutions. If you overeat at buffets, limit your portion size and just taste. If you overeat at parties, eat something before you go so you will not feel famished and can concentrate on talking to people.

◆ Limit alcohol intake, which can lower your resistance to problem foods and influence food choices.

Eliminate Guilt and Depriving Yourself

◆ The more extreme and restrictive a food plan is, the harder it is to follow.

◆ Depriving yourself causes fatigue and lowered athletic performance.

◆ Allow yourself to have small portions of food you like on a regular basis.

◆ Eliminate the guilt you may associate with eating.

Go Slowly and Reward Yourself

◆ Remember that effective weight loss and reduction of body fat occur slowly.

◆ Set achievable short-term goals along the way.

◆ Celebrate your victories by doing something positive: buy a new CD, wear clothes that you like, or splurge for a manicure or pedicure when you meet your goals.

Table 1.2	

Ineffective Techniques for Losing Weight

Technique	Result
Skipping a meal	Hunger, then overeating later
Eliminating fat	Lack of vitamins, lack of full feeling, may lead to overeating later
Increasing exercise	May not compensate for food eaten, injury risk from overtraining, stress fracture, burnout
Limiting calories to 1,000 a day	Inadequate for daily life, results in lowered metabolic rate and muscle loss

Think about the techniques that you have used for losing weight. List those techniques here:

_____

_____

Weight Fluctuations

Rapid, frequent fluctuations in weight—such as a weight change of five or more pounds a week—can also be a concern. Such fluctuations are often accompanied by changes in performance, mood swings, and food cravings. If you have this problem, it can be related to several underlying medical conditions. See your doctor for a screening evaluation of menstrual weight gain, premenstrual syndrome, thyroid problems, and disordered eating practices (see chapter 2 for more information on disordered eating). The medical staff can do the screening and then refer you to a nutritionist and possibly a counselor. If you have big changes in appetite, establishing a daily food plan to avoid hunger and food cravings is part of the treatment. If you have premenstrual syndrome, eating regular meals, exercising, reducing stress, and sometimes using B vitamin supplements can help.

Some people have difficulty managing their weight because there is an emotional component to their eating patterns. Many of us turn to food when we are under stress, bored, studying or working, or tired. Keeping a daily diary of your moods and recognizing emotional triggers to eating can be helpful (see food diary, page 62). Then you can work on strategies to offset these triggers, such as replacing eating with something that really reduces stress. This can be a big step toward controlling overeating. If you are starving yourself and, then overeating when overwhelmed by hunger or stress, you could be on the road to bulimia. Recognizing the early warning signs and establishing a regular eating pattern can prevent mood swings, weight fluctuation, and the development of a serious eating problem (see chapter 3 for information about anorexia and chapter 4 for information about bulimia). Determine your daily energy needs (see chapter 5, page 128) and choose a diet plan to meet them. Make your goal learning to eat appropriately for your activity level and for your health, and eliminate weight fluctuations.

Reshaping Your Body Image to Prevent the Triad

In addition to a healthy diet, it is important to develop a positive body image. This is critical to your self-esteem and confidence, two factors that impact performance much more than an extra pound or two. Many girls and women wake up each morning feeling like failures because they do not look like the idealized women in print and film. They may step on a scale, and if they have not lost weight, they feel depressed. These feelings of low self-esteem, and thoughts such as, "All would be well if only I could lose some weight," lead people into extreme diets and disordered eating practices. These practices often do not result in effective weight control but rather a roller-coaster ride of mood and weight swings. Overcoming these problems can involve improving your body image and self-esteem and learning what is good and healthy about your body.

> *I love the way I feel and look after exercising hard. Even though I am sweaty and panting, I feel great and like I am on a natural high. I used to be sort of skinny, but now I have muscles and definition. I met my boyfriend after one of my hardest runs when I was completely wiped out, but feeling good. He said he was attracted to me by how happy and healthy I looked. Now we work out together and have a great time.*
>
> Laura, a sports marketing intern in New York City

Body Image Exercise

As you think about your body, try the following exercise. It might reveal a few things to you. First, write down how you feel about your body: Is it normal weight, slightly overweight, very overweight, or underweight? How do you feel about your height? On a sheet of paper, draw a picture of your body without any clothes. You don't have to be an artist or even artistically inclined to do this. Don't worry; your drawing need not be perfect or even realistic. In fact, the more free-form your drawing is, the better. It is an exercise to get at what you think and feel about your body. So pick up a pencil and draw yourself.

What do you see in this drawing? What does it look and feel like to you? What body parts do you like and dislike? What parts did you feel anxious about drawing or want to hide? Do you think anyone who knows you, like your best friend, will recognize you? Are there parts of your body that you distorted because you dislike them so much?

When girls and women in developed societies draw pictures of themselves, they usually feel dislike for many body parts and may even draw distorted images of parts of their bodies. They may draw their thighs large, even grotesquely large. Why? Because often, these body parts are the ones that we see first and see with a great deal of dislike. When we draw a picture of them, we distort them. We may also spend a lot of time focusing on the body parts we do not like, to the point where it can ruin our day. Sound familiar?

Body Image Challenge

The body parts that girls and women most commonly dislike and distort are the hips and thighs. Up to 90 percent of all women dislike their thighs, and 80 percent dislike their hips. What does your drawing show about these parts of your body?

Remember that Mother Nature designed us to have full, rounded hips and thighs, the better to carry sex-specific fat for that all-important function, childbearing. Fat is naturally stored in the hips and thighs for use during pregnancy and breast feeding. "Wait a minute," you say, "that's not where I want my body fat to be." Unfortunately, that is the way it is. You may have many concerns and worries about it, and you may try to eliminate your unwanted thigh fat, but it is a battle against your own biology—against the beautiful body you are meant to have.

In addition to enlarging and distorting disliked body parts, most women do not recognize their beautiful body parts. They do not draw their beautiful eyes; straight, white teeth; long, tapered fingers; or graceful neck. Where does this distorted body image come from? Again, we are taught from an early age to want to look like the unrealistically thin models portrayed in magazines and movies.

◇ Do You Have a Healthy Body Image?

Do you praise your strong muscles or curse every curve? Take this quiz to find out if they way you feel about your appearance is harmful to your health.

1. How many times a week do you weigh yourself? a. 7 (or more) b. 1 to 3 c. 0

2. The last time you grabbed a part of your body, and said, "Look at this fat" to someone was: a. a few weeks ago. b. just this morning. c. never.

3. Which of these things have you tried in order to lose weight? a. Thigh creams b. Weird contraptions that "massage" fat away c. Cutting some fat out of your diet d. Cutting all fat out of your diet e. "Miracle" supplements such as chromium picolinate f. Regular exercise g. A crash diet

4. You're getting ready to go out with your best friend. You tried on a pair of pants and she frowns at you disapprovingly. You vow to get: a. new pants. b. a new best friend. c. a new butt.

5. When you look in the mirror during an aerobics class, you think: a. I'm such a klutz. Next time I'll stand in the back. b. My arms are getting stronger from all the push-ups I've been doing. c. Everyone in this class is skinnier than me.

6. When you think of getting pregnant, you think: a. Boy, am I going to look fat. b. Boy, am I going to be excited. c. Both

7. Complete this sentence: Models are _____.

   a. freaks of nature—only 1 percent of the population. b. blessed with great genes. c. the paragon of female beauty, one I can achieve if only I try hard enough.

8. You go to the store to buy jeans. On the dressing room you discover that you need a size larger than you did last season. You: a. think, "This designer must have cut her jeans small." b. get depressed and leave the store with out trying anything else on. c. buy last season's size even if they're snug—you'll make them fit somehow.

9. How often do you think about your body? a. Almost never b. Whenever you pass your reflection in the mirror c. Day and night

10. True or false: You have clothes in your closet that are at least two sizes too small.

11. True or false: More than one of your close friends has an eating disorder.

12. True or false: You sometimes call yourself weight-related names (e.g., Tub-o-Lard, Hippo) out loud or just in your head.

13. You're planning a getaway to the Caribbean. What will you be wearing when you hit those white, sandy beaches? a. A bikini b. A simple one-piece swimsuit with a skirt and matching coverup that covers a lot c. A one-piece tank swimsuit

14. How would you feel after finishing a candy bar? a. I must go to the gym immediately and run at least three miles. b. One candy bar's not going to kill me—or my diet. c. Well, I blew it. Might as well polish off the leftover pizza in the fridge.

Scoring

1. a. *0* b. *1* c. *2*; **2.** a. *1* b. *0* c. *2*; **3.** a. *0* b. *0* c. *2* d. *1* e. *0* f. *2* g. *0*; **4.** a. *2* b. *1* c. *0*; **5.** a. *1* b. *2* c. *0*; **6.** a. *0* b. *2* c. *1*; **7.** a. *2* b. *1* c. *0*; **8.** a. *2* b. *0* c. *1*; **9.** a. *2* b. *1* c. *0*; **10.** T. *0* F. *2*; **11.** T. *0* F. *2*; **12.** T. *0* F. *2*; **13.** a. *2* b. *0* c. *1*; **14.** a. *1* b. *2* c. *0*

Analysis

21 to 31 points: Strong, sexy, and self-confident. In rare moments you might hate a particular part of your anatomy, but overall you have a very healthy body image. You don't play cruel tricks on yourself, like buying clothes a size or two too small or pre-setting your scale up a few pounds—you're too happy with your body for those mind games. You know that your body is much more that just looks; it's capable of amazing things from running a 5 km race to enjoying the sensuous pleasure of massage. "The ability to love your body doesn't depend on physical perfection," notes Adrienne Ressler, body image specialist at the Renfrew Center in Fort Lauderdale Florida. "It has more to do with having high self-esteem and being realistic about the body you've biologically inherited." Your mission: Spread the love-your-body vibes so all women can be as confident as you are.

10 to 20 points: You're OK, your body's OK. Half the time you appreciate your unique shape; but just as often, you rebel against your body. What's your best weapon on those days when your self-image is less than stellar? Your brain. "It's easy to start believing something when you hear it all the time," says Ressler. Remind yourself how great you can look whenever you start having self-denigrating thoughts. Even if you don't believe it at first," Ressler says, "keep doing it. Eventually you will."

(continued)

Do you have a healthy body image? *(continued)*

0 to 9 points: Call 1-800 HLP MY BOD. Your negative attitude about your body is detrimental to your self-esteem and happiness. Obsessively checking yourself in the mirror, resorting to dangerous weight loss scams, and otherwise berating your body will not make you look better. It's certain to make you feel worse. "You'll be miserable until you realize that your self-worth can't and shouldn't be weighed on the scale," says Ressler. Women with poor body images sometimes flock together, so evaluate if your friends also have a negative feelings about their bodies. If so, consider developing relationships with people who appreciate the more significant inner qualities that make you the unique woman you are. But don't leave it up to your friends—body love has to start with you. Consider talking about your body image with someone you trust to gain some needed perspective.

Reprinted, by permission, from S. Solin, 1997, "Do you have a healthy body image?" *Fitness* October, pp. 94-97.

New Body Image Approach

Very little emphasis is placed on helping young girls and women develop a positive body image. So we have to reverse years of focusing on disliked body parts. Try this exercise. Close your eyes, and mentally list what you think of as your good points (they are the parts of your body and face that get compliments and that you like). Keep going until you have listed at least five things you like or have been admired for. Now, write those down.

Next, come up with some ideas for emphasizing those good parts. You may resolve to accentuate your eyes and eyebrows with a small amount of makeup or to spend time taking care of your fingernails instead of looking in the mirror at your hips. One of the points of this exercise is to encourage you to avoid looking at those body parts you do not like and to appreciate those parts you are happy with. Do not squeeze your thighs and look for cellulite! Instead, concentrate on your beautiful hair, your strong arms, or great smile. Come up with your own plan to emphasize the positive and to stop focusing on the negative.

In this chapter, we have reviewed the reasons women feel pressure to lose weight, push themselves into dieting, and try to attain unrealistic bodies. We have given you methods for effective weight control and building a positive body image. In the chapters that follow, we will show you how to recognize and avoid the pitfalls of disordered eating (anorexia and bulimia), amenorrhea, and osteoporosis.

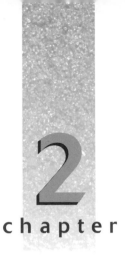

chapter

Thin Is In:
Disordered Eating

In chapter 1 we learned about some of Western society's ideal body images and how those preferred shapes have changed over the years. We also saw how misguided training practices can encourage athletic women to be unrealistically thin—too thin to win. This thin-equals-fit, lose-weight attitude is promoted in magazines and on television as well as by some coaches, trainers, parents, and even athletes themselves. It is not a healthy attitude, especially for hardworking, physically active women. To perform your best physically and mentally, you need a strong, muscular, well-fed body, not a starved, gaunt one.

However, because of external pressures and their own desire to be thin, many women turn to dieting as a means of slimming down. This chapter addresses the no-win situation that chronic dieting leads to and explains how such attempts affect performance and health in a negative way. Chronic dieting not only creates an energy deficit but also leads to the serious disorders of the female athlete triad. The end result is usually a loss of muscle and strength, not fat, and can include a wide range of unhealthy side effects that may require medical treatment.

At first, a woman may think, "Hey, I'm losing weight and I'm do-ing better in my sport!" This leads her to think, "If I lose more weight, I might be even better." She will reach a point where the energy deficit from dieting or disordered eating practices begins to harm her performance in several ways.

In the short term, reduced food intake impairs muscle recovery and rebuilding after exercise. The dieting athlete often does not store enough glycogen (carbohydrate) to fuel her muscles for the next workout. Low glycogen stores will cause her performance to drop considerably after about 30 minutes of exercise. Low protein intake causes the body to break down muscle tissue in order to get the amino acids it needs to make new cells.

Additionally, using diuretics and laxatives, vomiting, and fasting can lead to dehydration and lack of normal electrolytes like sodium and potassium. The result can be muscle cramps and loss of coordi-nation and balance. If you are 1 percent dehydrated, your performance decreases 2 to 3 percent. For example, in one study a well-hydrated athlete ran the mile in 7:00. She was then artificially dehydrated by 1 percent in a sauna, and her mile time increased to 7:40.

In the long term, you may not have enough calcium to build bone and you'll be at risk for stress fractures. Chronic undernourishment leads to loss of muscle tissue, injuries that don't heal, and heartbeat irregularities. You are also not providing enough fuel for your brain, so concentration and memory may suffer, resulting in moodiness and irritability.

We already know who is at risk—active women of nearly every age. Whether you're a competitive athlete or an active woman who just wants to be fit and healthy, there are steps you can take to avoid disordered eating habits. By understanding why dieting and disordered eating practices don't work, you can avoid them and perform your best.

Faced with the pervasive pressures to be lean and thin, and often dissatisfied with her own body shape, what's a woman to do? If she is like most of her friends, she learns about dieting. Americans spend $33 billion a year on weight loss products and services. Mothers teach their daughters dieting habits or put their daughters on diets, particularly during the later stages of puberty, when the female hor-mones create hips, breasts, and thighs. Mothers see their daughter's bodies changing and may believe the girls are getting fat. At an early age, girls also learn from hearing adult women talking about dissatisfaction with their body images. Comments from fathers, brothers, and boyfriends can also affect girls. A single off-the-cuff comment from an uninformed coach, trainer, or teammate can start a girl scrutinizing her body and coming to hate things about it. By the time girls are in high school, most have been on a diet or are currently dieting (see figure 2.1).

A 1996 survey of Australian girls ages 14 to 17 reported that 63 percent thought they were overweight, even though only 16 percent were (slightly) overweight. Forty-seven percent were dieting and 33 percent had disordered eating practices. Their dieting was motivated by peer pressure and media images (Grigg 1996).

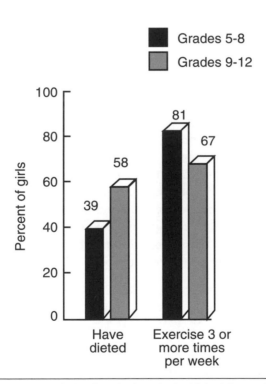

Figure 2.1 A Commonwealth Fund study done in the United States showed that girls in grades 5-8 were more likely to exercise and less likely to diet than girls in grades 9-12. The survey also found that 13 percent of the younger girls and 18 percent of the older girls reported regular binge and purge episodes.

Reprinted, by permission, from J.E. Meyer, J.M. Leiman, N. Rothschild, and M. Falik, 1999, "Improving the health of adolescent girls," *Policy Report of the Commonwealth Fund Commission on Women's Health*, January: 10.

Veronica, a 20-year-old student, had been dieting since she was in grade school. Her mother told her she came from a family of overweight women who gained weight in their thighs over the years. With very little success, the women in Veronica's family tried each new diet fad or book that came along. Veronica was physically active in high school, on the swim team and cheerleading squad, and she was always dieting to fit into her swimsuit. On entering college at a school 1,000 miles away from home, she found it hard to control her eating in the dorm, especially during midterms and finals. Much to her mother's dismay, she gained 10 pounds by the winter holidays of her freshman year. Her mother gave her a new diet book and cans of diet drinks and told her to get control of herself. Veronica had planned to try out for the swim team, but she now felt too fat to even put on the sleek swimsuits she had worn in high school. She tried living on the diet drinks for a few days, but she felt tired and irritable and ended up eating late-night pizza with her dorm mates. Fearful about going home overweight at spring break, she joined the campus fitness center to take some aerobics classes and lose a few pounds. She had always enjoyed the great feeling she got after a workout. Now she wanted to lose some weight and tone her hips, thighs, and abs. She hoped she could lose 20 pounds and would never have to diet again. She put a poster on her refrigerator of an elite Olympic athlete in a high-cut swimsuit diving into a pool. She started going to the gym seven days a week and restricted her calorie intake to 1,200 calories a day.

DO DIETS WORK?

Most of us have been on a diet at one time or another. You know the routine. You think you have to lose some weight, and you want to lose it fast and see the results. Full of enthusiasm, you start a diet, choosing something that seemed to work before or the latest fad from a magazine or book. Within a few days, you find that the weight is not rolling off as fast as you expected, and you feel frustrated and discouraged, not to mention hungry.

Feeling that the diet is not working, you might give it up altogether, turn to a more stringent diet, begin to exercise more intensely, or start cheating. Because a diet deprives your body of the fuel and nutrition it

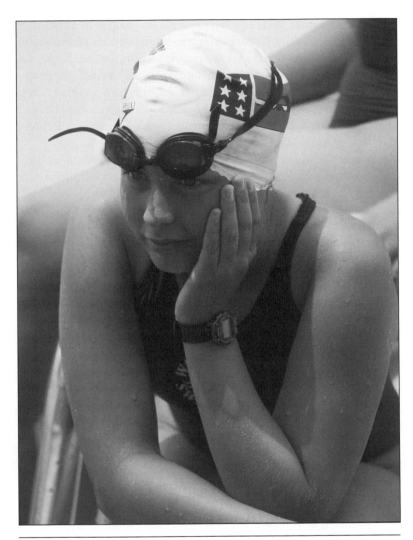

Your body cannot perform at its best while it is struggling with the low glyco-gen stores, low protein intake, and slow metabolic rate that accompany dieting.

needs to function at its best—and certainly to push itself in training and exercise—it is doomed to fail. Physiologically, your body interprets dieting as semistarvation. That is, when you cut calories and skip meals, your body slows down its metabolic rate to protect itself from famine and starvation.

Diets fail because they make you hungry. In response, you overeat, in spite of all your will power. Most people cannot stay on diets for long because of their natural "hunger hormones"—epinephrine, glucagon, and cortisol—which surge during times of reduced food intake. The hunger hormones alert your brain to search for food and to wolf down anything that is available. These hormones have powerful effects on your body and mood. Epinephrine (also known as adrenaline) is not only a hunger hormone but also is the hormone of the fight-or-flight response. It can make you feel jittery, irritable, anxious, and hungry. You can go on an emotional roller-coaster ride of highs and lows because of these hunger hormones. Know the feeling? You have been dieting all day, then you ravenously eat something forbidden and "blow your diet."

These hormones also function to break down the body's stored energy (stored as glycogen and fat) and to find amino acids (the building blocks of protein) for new cells. Your body needs protein to make new hair, skin, muscle, and other cells every day. Your body has no ability to store protein. If you do not eat enough on a daily basis, the hunger hormones will break down your body's own protein—primarily muscle—to make the necessary new cells. When you diet and go into a calorie deficit—burning more calories than you take in—you break down glycogen (also known as carbohydrate) and protein from muscle before you start to lose fat.

Thus, the best plan for healthy and effective weight control is to slightly reduce your daily caloric intake (by 200 to 300 calories) and to exercise regularly (see the sidebar on pages 28–30). Successful weight control involves keeping some changes in lifestyle after the diet is over so that the unwanted weight does not return. But even with the careful supervision and guidance from doctors and nutritionists, most people regain the weight they lose on a diet. Why? Remember the set point from chapter 1 (page 24). After a diet, your body is programmed to return to its genetically programmed, healthy weight.

> Like most of us, **Veronica** found it difficult to stick to a strict diet. She tried to eat very little all day, and drank Diet Coke to blunt her appetite. By 4 P.M., during her last class, she felt tired and had trouble concentrating. She often had to borrow a friend's notes because she had missed major points of the lecture. She felt famished afterward and occasionally found herself putting coins into a vending machine and eating junk food. Feeling guilty, she went to work out with a vengeance and vowed to start her diet anew the next day.

Your Body's Response to Dieting

Your metabolic rate is the number of calories that you burn when you are going about your normal day-to-day activities. Most women have a resting metabolic rate of 1,200 to 1,800 calories a day depending on their age, activity level, and body composition. As a result of dieting (lowering the number of calories your body takes in every day), your body slows down its metabolic rate and you do not burn as many calories. After repeated episodes of dieting, it takes longer for your metabolic rate to recover its normal rate. This slower metabolic rate in chronic dieters is the reason some women find they eat very little but do not lose weight.

You diet because you want to lose fat. As previously mentioned, during most diets, you lose muscle and stored carbohydrate (glycogen) before you lose fat. When weight is regained, as it often is in chronic dieters, much of the gain is in the form of fat (figure 2.2). After each episode of dieting and subsequent weight gain, you end up with less lean muscle mass and a greater body fat percentage. Muscle may weigh slightly more than fat, but it also burns more calories at rest. The lowered amount of muscle (lean body) mass is the part of the reason for a lowered metabolic rate.

> **Veronica** enjoys the step aerobics classes and has added weight training twice a week and a spinning class to her workouts. She still wants to get in good enough shape to try out for the swim team and get into her bathing suit. She looks at her body several times a day, feeling disgusted by what she thinks is cellulite in her thighs. She can see something that looks like cellulite when she squeezes her thigh skin together and looks closely in the mirror. She is hungry after a workout, but she eats only a salad with low-fat dressing. Later, alone in her apartment, she finds herself famished before bedtime and often eats cookies, ice cream, or several bowls of cereal before bed. The food is something she knows she shouldn't be eating, but she is tired of not eating all day, and she is stressed about upcoming exams. Somehow eating makes her feel relaxed and able to sleep. The next day, she recommits to her workout program and promises to add some time on a stair climber to burn more fat. Veronica is now working out two to three hours a day and has no spare time to socialize. Her friends never see her.

The other bad news about dieting is that it leads to the kind of overeating Veronica experienced. She dieted and worked out all day, and then late in the day, feeling stressed out, she ate more than was on her diet for three days! Do you ever feel famished or deprived when you are on a diet?

Research About the Effects of Dieting

In the 1950s, it was well established that dieting is a precursor to disordered eating practices and a distorted self-image. Studies by Ancel Keys and associates at the University of Minnesota evaluated the effects of a semistarvation, 1,800-calorie-per-day diet on 36 healthy young men. These men developed many of the disordered eating practices now reported in women who chronically diet. The men were preoccupied with thoughts of food, hoarded food, excessively chewed gum, and consumed coffee or tea. On their small daily food ration they ate voraciously, to the point of feeling bloated and uncomfortable. Some men self-induced vomiting to rid themselves of this bloated feeling. Many felt anxious or depressed. They reported being embarrassed and guilty about their supposed overeating behavior. One man shoplifted food and others had significant mood swings. Many became withdrawn, isolated, and experienced a decrease in sexual interest. The physical changes included a 40 percent decrease in basal metabolic rate, dizziness, headache, hair loss, decreases in strength, and tingling of hands and feet. This study demonstrated that a semistarved state, brought on by chronic dieting, produces significant physical and psychological problems in men as well as women. It showed that dieting is one cause of disordered eating behaviors and that some psychological disorders are related to dieting.

Many people blow their diets by overeating at the end of a day or after being stimulated by a lot of food. Let's say that you are on a strict diet and try to eat in the dorm cafeteria, or you go to a party where everyone is eating. Without thinking about it, you go back for seconds in the cafeteria line or you eat a whole plate of appetizers. This rapid, almost unconscious, automatic eating is a response to the hunger hormones your body produces when deprived of food for hours; the hormones commanded you to eat. Veronica found that after a few days of her strict diet, she came home and ate a whole box of Fig Newtons. The men in the semistarvation study hoarded food, then gorged and felt bloated and guilty. A lot of calories can be consumed during this kind of automatic eating. Now you may understand why you sometimes have the urge to eat everything in sight after you have been dieting for several days.

An athletic woman needs more calories because of the demands that exercise puts on her body. Your body knows it needs more calories and will do almost anything to get them. You can suddenly eat

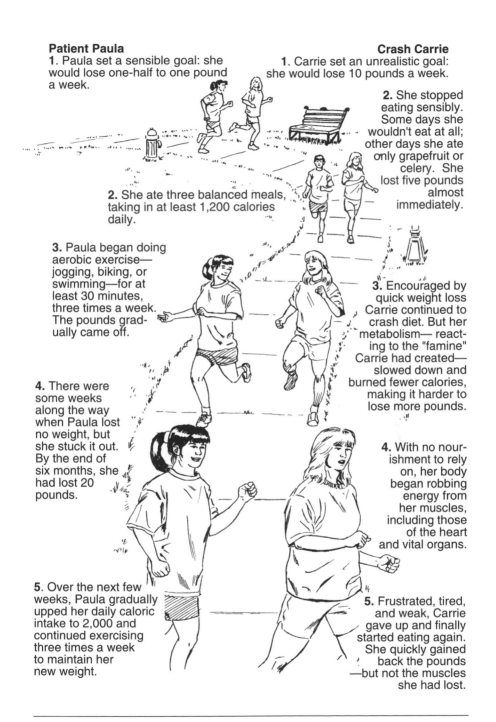

Patient Paula

1. Paula set a sensible goal: she would lose one-half to one pound a week.

2. She ate three balanced meals, taking in at least 1,200 calories daily.

3. Paula began doing aerobic exercise— jogging, biking, or swimming—for at least 30 minutes, three times a week. The pounds gradually came off.

4. There were some weeks along the way when Paula lost no weight, but she stuck it out. By the end of six months, she had lost 20 pounds.

5. Over the next few weeks, Paula gradually upped her daily caloric intake to 2,000 and continued exercising three times a week to maintain her new weight.

Crash Carrie

1. Carrie set an unrealistic goal: she would lose 10 pounds a week.

2. She stopped eating sensibly. Some days she wouldn't eat at all; other days she ate only grapefruit or celery. She lost five pounds almost immediately.

3. Encouraged by quick weight loss Carrie continued to crash diet. But her metabolism— reacting to the "famine" Carrie had created— slowed down and burned fewer calories, making it harder to lose more pounds.

4. With no nourishment to rely on, her body began robbing energy from her muscles, including those of the heart and vital organs.

5. Frustrated, tired, and weak, Carrie gave up and finally started eating again. She quickly gained back the pounds —but not the muscles she had lost.

Figure 2.2 Crash dieting and other restrictive dieting methods are not effective means of losing weight and becoming fit. A sensible, nutritious diet paired with consistent exercise is the most effective way to lose or maintain your weight while staying healthy.

more during automatic eating than you have eaten all day. The downfall of diets is that the body will do all it can to undermine them.

Your Emotions and Dieting

In our society, we do not consume food simply to get nutrients. We eat at times of celebration, when we mark special occasions, and as a reward for doing something well. Food is also very enjoyable. The taste of our favorite foods is a real delight. Certain foods have effects on brain chemistry and mood, as anyone who loves chocolate can tell you.

Some women use food as an antidote for depression or anger or as a temporary solution to loneliness. Eating can be a form of self-expression, and it can be a self-treatment for feelings of inadequacy or loss. When women overeat because they are lonely, stressed, or depressed, they feel ashamed, embarrassed, and guilty afterward. They then want to diet again or disgorge the food they just ate. This cycle of bulimic behavior is discussed in more detail in chapter 4.

Why Don't Diets Work?

Diets don't work for a number of reasons:

- It is hard to stay on them, because they are a form of restriction. Your mind and body rebel against not getting enough of the fuel they need.
- Diets often confuse and alter your metabolism by slowing it down.
- Diets change your body composition by lowering muscle and preserving fat.
- Almost all diets lead to overeating. Your body is programmed to return to its set point—the weight at which you are healthy.

DOES EXERCISE WORK?

Many of us enjoy the benefits of being physically active. Weight management and weight control are some of the benefits. Women who are physically active gain muscle and reduce body fat as a natural part of training. Physically active women have a higher resting metabolic rate and tend to have a greater sense of well-being than their non-exercising counterparts. Many exercisers get a long-lasting "workout high." However, our society pressures women not only to be fit and enjoy physical activity but also to be thin as a result of their exercise. For women, getting in shape often means getting thinner rather than developing cardiovascular fitness, muscle strength, flexibility, and endurance. This is much different from the "get fit" message many men hear, which emphasizes getting bigger and stronger.

Some women also use exercise to make up for not following their diets or for overeating. Cory, a patient I cared for over several years, had a strict diet program. If she strayed from her diet, she calculated how many calories she had overeaten, and she exercised to burn up those calories. Her life revolved around eating and then exercising to burn off what she ate. She would not go out with friends or enjoy a movie or concert if she "needed" to exercise. She lost the ability to have fun and to enjoy eating. Her boyfriend could no longer tolerate her obsession, and he broke up with her. While she carefully calculated calories, she did not count on the price her social life and body would have to pay for this obsession. She eventually developed a stress fracture that made it painful to exercise.

Cory came to see me after this injury and asked for a diet that would increase her metabolic rate so that she would not gain weight. I advised her to relax the tight dieting and the over-exercising so that her body could heal and return to a normal metabolic rate. At first Cory did not believe me. I referred her to a nutritionist and psychologist. Over the next six months, we saw her frequently. She was able to increase her calcium and protein intake and her stress fracture healed in three months. It took her longer to reestablish a normal relationship with food.

Long-term studies of normal-weight people have shown that exercise programs alone can reduce body weight by about 5 percent. Exercise by itself is usually not enough to lead a woman to an unrealistic level of extreme thinness. Combining diet and exercise is generally the best method for slow, sustained weight loss. Gradual weight loss and firming of muscles is exactly what happens in athletic training. It happens slowly, and you should not expect to lose more than one-half to one pound a week during exercise training or even when dieting alone.

The main reason not to lose weight too quickly is that your energy level, performance, and training will all suffer. If you try to lose weight faster than a rate of about a one pound a week, you will break down muscle, which is a definite detriment for an athletic woman. Losing too much weight too fast creates other medical problems, as well. You may become dehydrated and fatigued, both of which drastically reduce your performance and increase your risk for injury. Losing weight too quickly can also cause existing injuries to not heal effectively and can result in low blood sugar levels, decreasing concentration and coordination.

Like Veronica, many women combine a strict diet with heavy exercise in an attempt to lose weight as fast as possible. However, aside from the detriments to your energy levels and athletic performance already mentioned, the energy drain may be great enough that your body shuts down other systems to conserve; you may stop having menstrual cycles (see chapter 5), which can then lead to stress fractures in the short term and osteoporosis later in life (see chapter 6).

WHEN DOES DIETING BECOME DISORDERED EATING?

When a diet doesn't seem to work, or work fast enough, many people get desperate and frustrated. They turn to even stricter diets, start using diuretics (substances that cause the body to rid itself of water) or diet pills, or experiment with self-induced vomiting. Other behaviors might include food fadism (choosing to eat only selected food groups or following fad diets), fasting, forcing oneself to vomit, using saunas to sweat off weight, spitting out food that has been chewed, and using laxatives and even enemas. Most of us know people who have tried to lose weight in one of these ways. What most people do not know is that *these techniques do not work*. They cause loss of water weight, not fat weight, and they have significant medical and psychological side effects (see table 2.1). Such practices can be classified as disordered eating practices, harmful eating behaviors that do not result in true weight loss.

Usually, the first signs of the female athlete triad are seen in women using these practices. Disordered eating—as opposed to clinically defined eating disorders—covers a wide spectrum of behaviors. Some people may use one of these techniques occasionally. Others may experiment with many different techniques frequently, as often as several times a day. What may start as a desire and a means to drop a few pounds can eventually lead to a full-blown eating disorder. If left unrecognized or untreated, disordered eating can cause irregular menstrual cycles, another symptom of the triad. Although not all diets develop into disordered eating, most eating disorders begin with a "harmless" diet. Veronica is a case in point.

Frustrated at not losing weight, **Veronica** started a new restrictive diet. She didn't realize or remember that she was hungry most of the time and overeating at night on her previous diet. Instead of starting the day with a low-fat, high-protein breakfast that would curb her hunger and give her energy, she completely skipped breakfast, because that is when her willpower was highest. She began to weigh herself several times a day and felt like a failure if she had not lost weight. One day she gained a pound after eating a small lunch of frozen yogurt, Diet Coke, and an apple. Her stomach seemed to her to be huge and bloated. She remembered a pill advertised in a woman's magazine to treat "that bloated feeling." She bought some of these pills over the counter at a drugstore. This pill is a diuretic, which forces water out of the body by causing the kidneys to produce more urine. After taking twice the recommended dose, she was up several times in the night going to the bathroom. Veronica noticed that although she didn't sleep well, she lost two pounds overnight. This was not a loss in real body weight, just water, and along with it, essential electrolytes. She was dehydrated and she did not perform her best, doing poorly on some midterms. She was also dizzy during her workouts.

Such practices may make it appear that you lose weight in the short term, but you do not lose the dreaded body fat. These practices cause dehydration. After all, the human body is 70 percent water. You can get a great deal of weight change overnight, if you lose some of the body's water. Along with the loss of body water, these methods also drain you of essential electrolytes that regulate the electrical and chemical balance among nerves, muscles, and fluids. Electrolytes also control the electrical activity and contraction of muscles, including the heart. The loss of fluids and electrolytes can lead to serious medical problems in addition to dehydration, including acid base abnormalities and heart irregularities. The result is lightheadedness, muscle cramps, skipped or irregular heartbeats, gastrointestinal problems, and even fainting. Dehydration and electrolyte abnormalities can further be detrimental to physical activity by decreasing coordination, balance, and muscle function.

Table 2.1

Consequences of Disordered Eating Practices

Practice	Consequence
Fasting	Loss of lean body mass (muscle), lowered metabolic rate
Diet pills	Anxiety, rapid heartbeat, weight regained quickly, high blood pressure
Diuretics (water pills)	Dehydration, no fat loss, abnormal electrolytes
Laxatives	Diarrhea, dehydration, abdominal pain, dependency
Sauna	Dehydration, no fat loss
"Fat-free" diet	Lack of vitamins, lack of satiety (fullness), hard to follow
Excessive exercise	Risk of injury
Enemas	Dehydration
Self-induced vomiting	Dehydration, abnormal acid-base balance, electrolyte abnormalities, erosion of dental enamel, bleeding from stomach, tears of esophagus

---

Disordered eating practices are not as serious as the eating disorders bulimia and anorexia. However, they are a first step on the road to developing eating disorders and the female athlete triad. Many women experiment with these practices and then begin using them on a regular basis. Before long, they may find their lives start to revolve around the use of laxatives or vomiting after meals. Once the use becomes a regular pattern for three months or more, a woman has developed a clinically defined eating disorder (in this example, bulimia; see chapter 4).

Veronica lost eight pounds in two weeks with her strict dieting, exercising, and occasional use of diuretics. She felt great in her tightest jeans and felt okay in a high-cut swimsuit. She thought if she just lost five more pounds she would be ready to try out for the swim team. She wanted to go home for summer break thinner than ever and show her mom how disciplined she was. However, she was irritable a lot of the time, and her friends commented on how they never saw her anymore. A few times she had felt lightheaded, and she had almost passed out once when she was lifting weights. Trying to lose the last five pounds, she experimented with diet pills to stop her hunger. One night, after she had "overeaten" by having two bowls of cereal for dinner, she felt extremely bloated. The diuretic did not make her feel thin enough, so she took several laxatives. During the night and the next morning, she had painful stomach cramps and diarrhea, and she doubled over in pain during her morning class. One of her friends saw her and insisted she go to the Student Health Center for a checkup. I was the doctor on duty, and when I took a history, I realized Veronica was in the throes of a serious eating disorder.

Food fads are diet plans that do not provide balanced nutrition or adequate energy. A person who follows one food fad or diet after another may be struggling with disordered eating or body image issues. As anyone who has lived with a teenager knows, food fads can be part of adolescence. The struggle for independence often takes the form of very selective eating—vegetarianism, no red meat, and "fat-free" diets are common. But many adults try food fads as well, such as very low-calorie liquid or protein diets that do not meet their basic metabolic needs.

Susan was an apple-cheeked, bouncy 13-year-old who started a diet when she went to a new school in seventh grade. She was teased by the ninth-grade boys for being "fat" and having chipmunk cheeks (she had inherited her round cheeks from her dad). She was not overweight at all, but the teasing made her feel fat. First she started cutting out all desserts and butter. She found that most of the girls at school did not bring lunch, but instead ate a salad or skipped lunch, and she started doing this as well. She stopped eating red meat and cut all the fat off of chicken. She insisted that her mother buy only fat-free food. She decided to become a vegetarian after one of her new friends told her she could really lose weight by not eating meat.

Many women avoid whole classes of foods in an effort to have a fat-free diet. They may almost completely eliminate dairy products and meat because these are regarded as fattening. And yet, these are the food groups that contain iron and calcium—the minerals and vitamins essential to the health and growth of young women. Adolescent girls need nearly twice the calcium and iron that boys need, and adult women need more than adult men. (For more detailed information on calcium needs and how to meet them, see chapter 6.)

Foods labeled fat-free are sought after as though they were treasures to hoard. In fact, many of these foods are actually quite high in calories from carbohydrates and sugar, and these are converted to fat by the liver if there is an excess. That means if you don't use the carbohydrate or sugar—ready-to-use energy—the body stores it as fat. There are some other potential problems with very-low-fat diets. They can be deficient in fat-soluble vitamins (A, E) and can lead to impaired growth of cell membranes. The fat-soluble vitamins are crucial to athletic women, whose bodies are necessarily in a constant process of breaking down and rebuilding muscle, bone and other cells. Low-fat diets cause dry skin and brittle hair and increase your hunger. Without fat in the diet to give you the sense of pleasant fullness known as satiety, your body craves more food. An hour or more after you eat, you may feel hungry again. The lack of satiety from the low-fat diet then leads to increased hunger and overeating.

WHO IS AT RISK?

You can often predict which girls and women will develop disordered eating patterns and subsequent eating disorders. Models, entertainers, beauty pageant contestants, and athletes who have to wear skimpy outfits are at an increased risk for turning to these seemingly quick-fix but actually dangerous techniques. Women with certain lifestyles, or those who participate in activities that emphasize a lean appearance, have weight categories, or mandate weigh-ins (for example, women in the military and athletes in sports like gymnastics, figure skating, rowing, martial arts, cheerleading, baton twirling, and the like), are at more risk. Some athletic women are told they will be faster, will jump higher, or will perform better if they lose weight.

Adolescents

The changes in a girl's body at the time of puberty (see chapter 1), coupled with peer pressure, make adolescence the most vulnerable time. Whereas a boy gains more muscle and grows taller and leaner at puberty, a girl gains fat for reproductive functioning. The natural process of development is working for the survival of the species. Women who try to lose their female body fat are fighting a battle of evolutionary proportions. Just when girls are desperate to be slim and attractive, their body fat percentages increase. Boys value the body changes that occur during puberty to make them stronger, faster, and larger. Girls do not value their body changes, because our society has rejected the fertile (fat) female body as the ideal.

Laura was a budding gymnast who had loved the sport since she was four years old, when she first saw Olympic gymnastics. Her parents paid for private lessons, and she competed on a local club team. When she was 12, she started going through the changes of puberty, developing breasts and becoming taller. Her club gymnastics coach told her that if she didn't stop growing or gaining weight, "it was all over" for her as a gymnast and that it was unlikely she would ever get a college scholarship, much less a shot at the Olympics. She was told to go on a strict diet, and she was weighed daily before practice. In an effort to stop her body from growing, she lived on salads and fat-free yogurt, and she often found herself exhausted. In contrast, Laura's older brother was playing soccer, and at age 14, he was starting his growth spurt. He was urged by his coach to eat more, bulk up, and gain weight.

When I talked to **Veronica** in the student health clinic, she told me she was on a strict diet to lose "the freshman 10 pounds." Like many young women starting a new phase in life, Veronica's lifestyle and eating patterns had changed. She found that she handled some of the stress of college by snacking and ordering pizza. Alarmed at her weight gain, she desperately tried to lose weight in order to fit in and feel more attractive.

Women Under Stress and in Transition

Stressful periods of transition, such as beginning high school or college, starting a new job, having a baby, or moving to a new town, may put a woman at risk for disordered eating. Faced with a new environment, a woman may feel that the best way to be accepted or to succeed is to have the "right" appearance. Because being overly thin is currently considered ideal, losing weight is one way a woman can fit in, become popular, and handle uncertainty. In the case of postpregnancy, her motives might be to "get back to where she was" or "be sexy again for my husband."

Athletes

Several studies show that some athletes are at increased risk for disordered eating behaviors compared to nonathletic women. The increased risk is not due to being an athlete or participating in sports. Rather, it arises because of the pressure placed on some athletic women to lose weight.

We've seen that disordered eating practices and weight loss are harmful to athletes. We've also learned, in chapter 1, that being thinner does not necessarily lead to improved athletic performance. So, why would an athlete want to lose weight? As we've discussed, in addition to the general pressure women face, many athletes have the added pressure of misplaced emphasis on body weight and appearance as indicators or measures of success in their sports.

As the opportunities in women's sports have increased, so have the stakes. When the stakes go up, so do the pressures and the risks that people take to be successful. A young female athlete who has the right look and is successful can make money in endorsements, get a scholarship, or even win professional prize money.

Ellen, a member of her high school softball and volleyball teams, told us that most of

By talking to and supporting teammates who may be struggling with dieting or body image issues, athletes can help one another avoid the triad.

her volleyball teammates were dieting to get into their tight uniforms but that her softball teammates were much more relaxed about dieting. The sport or the exercise program itself is not the problem. As previously noted, it is the pressure to lose weight (which can be self-generated or exerted by coaches, families, and teammates) that is the problem. This pressure can set an athletic girl on the road to disordered eating and the female athlete triad. A remark by a coach that, "you'd be quicker on the court if you were lighter," or a comment about how a girl looks in a very skimpy outfit can start disordered eating behavior in girls and women. It takes a fair amount of self-esteem, self-acceptance, and a positive body image to become immune to these messages.

Some of the personality traits that make women successful athletes may place them at risk for disordered eating. These traits include heightened body awareness, a drive to succeed, perfectionism, self-discipline, compulsiveness, and self-control. An athlete's desire to excel at almost any cost, coupled with pressure from a coach to lose weight, can create a situation leading to disordered eating. Athletes are accustomed to working hard, living with pain, and denying themselves in the pursuit of excellence. Athletes live in a competitive culture in which diet and weight may be critically important to their appearance and performance. Athletes may compete among themselves to be not only the fastest or strongest but also the thinnest or most able to diet.

> *The very thing that makes a great athlete or a great student or a great businessperson already predisposes them to be obsessive. Add on top of that that the sport demands you to be young, demands you to be thin, and where perfection is the name of the game. . . . If she happens to have a coach that is demanding, that very thing that makes her coachable can lead to a problem.*
>
> Cathy Rigby, a two-time Olympic gymnast who was hospitalized twice during a 12-year battle with bulimia (*Newsday*, July 27, 1997)

Athletes at most risk for eating disorders are those whose inherited body types do not match the sport-related ideal. With raw physical talent and hard work, some elite athletes are able to overcome a body type that does not match the ideal. However, women who were not born with the ideal body try harder to get the edge that would make them the best. They are often wrongly told or erroneously believe that losing weight is the most important way to gain success. Thus, these sub-elite athletes may be at more risk for eating disorders than elite athletes are.

Research on Disordered Eating in Athletes

In a study of 182 females athletes at Midwestern universities, 32 percent admitted using disordered eating practices frequently (at least twice a week for at least one month). Twenty-four percent self-induced vomiting, and 16 percent used laxatives (Rosen, L., et.al. 1986). The athletes' reasons for using these techniques were as follows:

♦ To improve appearance (7 percent)

♦ To improve athletic performance (83 percent)

♦ Both reasons (10 percent)

Seventy percent of these athletes believed the techniques they were using were harmless.

A 1995 report surveyed 1,445 athletes at 10 American universities about risk factors for developing eating disorders (Johnston, 1997). The survey results showed that

♦ 58 percent of female and 38 percent of male athletes at these institutions were at risk for disordered eating practices;

♦ 19 percent of female athletes scored high on the body dissatisfaction index, and 16 percent scored high on the drive for thinness;

♦ 9 percent of female athletes and less than 1 percent of male athletes had disturbed eating behaviors that warranted clinical attention;

♦ 2 percent of the women had anorexia, and 4 percent had bulimia;

♦ the highest-risk sports were gymnastics and swimming for women and wrestling and gymnastics for men; and

♦ 23 percent of the female athletes had tried self-induced vomiting (7 percent reported this behavior monthly, 3 percent weekly, and 1.4 percent daily). Fourteen percent had used laxatives.

Many athletes, physicians, trainers, and athletic administrators have both horror stories and success stories about how coaches deal with their athletes' weight issues. One coach required all women who gained weight to run the stairs an additional 20 minutes after practices. It was no surprise that his team had high rates of stress fractures. One of the "overweight" athletes was a first-year student who was actually four months pregnant and too frightened to tell anyone. She ended up being benched by the coach because she did not lose weight.

Another coach required all athletes to be at 17 percent body fat before they were eligible to receive their varsity uniforms. This coach did not realize that the techniques used by her training room staff to measure body fat percentage were inaccurate, nor was she able to give a rationale for choosing the 17 percent figure. She was also not aware of the distress her athletes felt at having to be measured and having to hit the 17 percent mark. Many of her athletes used disordered eating practices before the body comp test. More coaching education about the role of nutrition in sport, body composition measurements, and normal weight and health in women is desperately needed (see chapter 8, page 250).

One of the best models for coaches is the one developed by Dr. Randa Ryan's Performance Team (University of Texas at Austin) (Ryan 1992, 1997). Refer back to figure 1.5 (page 26) for more details on that program. One key to the success of the program is education for athletes and coaches about nutrition, weight ranges, and risks of disordered eating. Medical professionals are included in a team approach that helps coaches deal with weight and weight control issues. The result is that athletes report less stress about weight issues. Eating disorders are preventable and treatable illnesses. It is critically important that coaches be involved in the prevention and treatment of these disorders.

PROTECTING YOURSELF AGAINST EATING DISORDERS

You can protect yourself against eating disorders. Knowledge is power and prevention is the best medicine. Knowing that disordered eating patterns don't work for effective weight management is the first step in avoiding them—and avoiding these behaviors is the best way to protect yourself from developing a full-blown eating disorder.

Joanne had been overweight as a preschooler. She started playing soccer when she was seven years old and soon lost her "baby fat." She joined a team and was one of the best midfield players. Her dad coached the team for a year, and her mom brought snacks of Fig Newtons, milk, fruit, and popcorn. The team took many trips together, and the girls all

(continued)

enjoyed team dinners of pizza and pasta. They did pancake breakfasts to raise money for travel. Joanne was proud of her strong legs and body. When she was 16, she told her mom that many of her friends at school were into weird diets. Most of her soccer teammates thought these diets were stupid. They knew they could eat normally and not worry about weight because they were athletic. Joanne tried to talk a few of her classmates into joining the team, but they didn't want to get "too muscular." Joanne and some of her teammates did a school project on good nutrition and put up posters about the USA gold-medal-winning World Cup and Olympic women's soccer teams. They banded together to resist the messages to diet and tried to influence the other girls at their school to have better self-images.

Disordered eating is common, complex, and preventable. Recognizing the behavior early is key to preventing a clinical eating disorder and developing the triad.

Are You at Risk for an Eating Disorder?

Mark the following statements true or false.

__ Even though people tell me I'm thin, I feel fat.

__ I get anxious if I can't exercise.

__ I worry about what I will eat.

__ If I gain weight, I get anxious or depressed.

__ I feel guilty when I eat.

__ I would rather eat by myself than with family or friends.

__ I don't talk about my fear of being fat, because no one understands how I feel.

__ I have a secret stash of food.

__ When I eat, I'm afraid I won't be able to stop.

__ I get anxious when people urge me to eat.

__ Sometimes I think that my eating or exercising is not normal.

Number of true statements

◆ 1 to 3: You have a mild preoccupation with weight and appearance. Reevaluate. Don't lose control.

◆ 4 to 6: There is reason for concern. Check with your doctor and an eating disorder specialist.

◆ 7 to 11: You are in danger. Make an appointment with your doctor.

Reprinted, by permission, from B. Ludovise, 1992, "Eating disorders: Toll on the body," *Los Angeles Times,* December 6. Copyright © *Los Angles Times Syndicate.*

Any person using disordered eating techniques can experience serious short- or long-term medical and psychological conditions identical to those seen in anorexia and bulimia: depression, low self-esteem, stomach and digestive problems, menstrual irregularities, heart problems, and even death by heart failure or suicide. Moreover, disordered eating practices are not going to help you excel in your sport—you'll become tired, dehydrated, and risk greater injuries if you don't provide your body with the energy it needs. Now that you understand the dynamics and dangers of disordered eating practices, you can help prevent their occurrence in your own life and the lives of your friends.

Veronica was frightened by the severity of her pain from using laxatives and having diarrhea all night. Fortunately, she was willing to talk about what was going on; many young women with disordered eating will do almost anything to keep it a secret. Veronica had had enough of the roller-coaster ride of dieting, diuretics, and overexercising that her life had become. Her grades were going down, and she was tired of being tyrannized by the number on her bathroom scale. Because of Veronica's willingness to get help, she was able to recover. She met with me, our school nutritionist, and a psychologist. The nutritionist helped her resume normal eating patterns so that she was not so hungry. The psychologist helped her with some of the issues with her family and her body image. She did gain back weight fairly quickly, but we reassured her that it was water weight and that she would settle down to a more stable weight within a few weeks.

Veronica began keeping a diary about her feelings, her food intake, and her exercise. She realized she often turned to food when she felt stressed, unhappy, or angry. With the help of the psychologist, she found other ways to express her feelings and stopped weighing herself. Six months later,

(continued)

Veronica was no longer using any disordered eating practices, was doing better in school, and had invited her mother to come to a family therapy session. Her mother became aware of how her pressure on Veronica to lose weight had contributed to the problem.

Veronica wasn't cured of her concerns about weight, but she was exercising for fun and health reasons. She decided not to join the swim team, but she enjoyed her aerobics classes and wanted to be a fitness instructor during summer breaks. Her relationship with her mother improved, and she continued in counseling. Her sophomore year she focused more on schoolwork, made more friends, and started dating. Her grades improved, and she found a steady boyfriend.

What Veronica Did Right

* Went for professional help
* Reestablished relationships with friends and family
* Stopped weighing herself
* Began a normal eating pattern—stopped dieting and using diuretics
* Worked to improve her body image and self-esteem
* Kept a diary about her feelings
* Learned to express her feelings in writing and by talking about them
* Began exercising for the fun of it; found she liked aerobics and gave up swimming
* Added stress busters—a yoga class and a relaxation tape
* Talked honestly with her mother about the pressure she felt

WHAT VERONICA'S EXPERIENCE TEACHES US

Veronica developed disordered eating behavior in a fairly typical way. If she'd recognized the early-warning signs and had taken action, she could have stopped before serious problems developed. If you notice these warning signs in yourself or someone else, there are many things you can do to prevent the development of disordered eating patterns.

Losing weight to improve performance

If you are told to lose weight by a coach to improve your performance, this should immediately send up a warning flag. Is this coach making a competent assessment? Or is it just a "gut feeling" on the coach's part?

Action to take: Concentrate on your training and technique. If you are not at the appropriate weight for your body and sport, dedicating yourself anew to the activity will bring this about in an appropriate way. Also, ask to see a nutritionist or medical professional so an expert can make the determination that you can safely lose weight and show you how to best go about it. Follow the guidelines in figure 1.5. Make sure you know how to properly fuel yourself for your sport.

Being pressured by others to lose weight

In Veronica's case, her mother pressured her to be thinner than was realistic for her body type. Pressure can come from many different sources and can make you feel unworthy.

Action to take: If you are getting pressure, tell the source to stop. Explain how upsetting it is to feel this pressure and how difficult it is to lose weight. Talk with whoever is pressuring you and decide to de-emphasize weight and emphasize health and fitness. If you have a medical or a legitimate performance reason to lose weight, do it in a slow, steady manner with professional support from a nutritionist.

Having unrealistic weight goals

Like many women, Veronica wanted to be an unrealistically low weight. Given her body build, it was not possible for her to lose 10 to 20 pounds. This thinking set her up for failure, because she felt she could never be thin enough. Striving to be unnaturally, impossibly thin leads directly to disordered behaviors such as vomiting and diuretics.

Action to take: If you have a weight loss goal, make sure it is reasonable and appropriate for your body build and for good health. Check in with either a nutritionist or medical professional, who can help you set a realistic timeline to lose weight with a combination of diet and exercise.

Participating in an activity that emphasizes a particular body type for success

Veronica was a cheerleader and swimmer, activities that can place a great deal of emphasis on being thin and that involve wearing body-revealing clothing.

Action to take: If your sport or activity requires you to change your body or to wear revealing clothing, decide if you can handle the pressure. If you decide to stay in this activity, choose to judge yourself by your performance, by your health, and by the way you meet your own goals. Don't compare yourself to others.

Using chronic dieting, fad diets, or fasting

Veronica had dieted all her life, and she was taught to do so by her mother. Dieting, restrictive food fads, and fasting can cause anyone to feel hungry and deprived. They lead to a lower resting metabolic rate and less muscle mass, and they often result in overeating. Chronic dieting has definitely been shown to lead to bingeing and then purging, the beginning of bulimia.

Action to take: Don't fall into the trap of starving yourself or following a restrictive fad diet. Consider keeping a food and mood diary following the template provided in table 2.2. Then, evaluate whether or not you need to lose weight at all. And if you decide you do need to lose, follow a reasonable, slow, steady weight-loss plan combined with your exercise program.

Table 2.2

Sample Daily Food and Mood Diary

Name: _____ Date: _____ Day of week: _____

Time of day	Location or activity	Foods eaten	Amount eaten (cups, ounces, etc.)	How prepared (boiled, etc.)?	No. of calories	Mood (happy, sad, bored, angry, etc.)

Turning to weight loss during times of stress or transitions

Like many of us, Veronica gained weight during a time of stress and change. Easy food access in the dorm and stopping her exercise contributed to her weight gain. Feeling uncertain in a new environment, Veronica thought that by losing weight she would be more self-confident, attractive, and successful. Instead, her dieting added to her stress.

Action to take: When you face a stressful time or a change, keep up your regular stress-management habits. Continue to exercise for your health and build in some new stress busters, such as relaxation, yoga, meditation, or spiritual practices. Seek advice on stress management from a counselor or psychologist. Don't be too hard on yourself, and find time to have fun and make friends.

Weighing or measuring yourself daily

Veronica determined how she felt about herself by the number on her scale. Over-attention to weight or emphasizing the size of your least-liked body part is a definite warning sign of body image problems and a recipe for unhappiness.

Action to take: Throw out the scale; stop looking at or measuring any body parts. Look at yourself as a whole person, and learn to accept who you are. Emphasize your positive body parts. Choose a part of your body you really like, and learn to enhance it.

Fighting with or withdrawing from friends and family

Veronica withdrew from her closest and most important relationships. She also did not make new friends. In isolation, her sense of self became more distorted and she became depressed. She thought the only way to be liked was to lose weight. Her life began to revolve around her eating behavior and sense of failure. Often, disordered eating is a symptom of disturbed relationships, depression, or low self-esteem.

Action to take: Don't lose touch with your friends, supporters, and family. They care for you whatever you weigh. Seek help from a counselor early if you have difficult relationships that contribute to your eating disorder or depression. Learn coping and communication skills that can help you express your feelings.

Overexercising

Veronica was exercising up to three hours a day. She gave up friends and studying. Her entire focus was limiting food and increasing exercise to lose weight. She had a compulsion to exercise and lost her enjoyment in working out. Anyone who does this is at high risk for injury, amenorrhea (see chapter 5), and burnout.

Action to take: If you are losing the joy of exercise, you are overdoing it. No one should work out seven days a week. Your body and mind need days off and days that are for fun and relaxation. Cut back, take a day off, change activities, do things with friends, and rediscover having fun with exercise instead of feeling driven to work out to burn off calories.

Using disordered eating practices

Veronica tried "quick-fix" techniques like diuretics to give the false appearance of weight loss. Weight that is lost quickly by dehydration is regained just as quickly.

Action to take: If you find you are using these techniques, *stop*. Use the information in this chapter to list reasons why you should stop. If you cannot stop on your own, *run*, don't walk, to seek medical and psychological help before you become addicted to these practices.

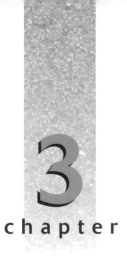

chapter

Dying To Be Thin: Anorexia Nervosa

We are very concerned about disordered eating habits because they can eventually lead to eating disorders. When a woman is suffering from a medically defined eating disorder, her life is dominated entirely by the disease. Of the two disorders, anorexia and bulimia, anorexia is the most dangerous, with a 15 to 18 percent death rate. In this chapter, we discuss the signs and symptoms of anorexia.

Chances are you know at least one person with this serious illness. As much as 1 to 2 percent of the young female population in the United States has anorexia. These women are likely to be among the brightest students, the best employees, and the "good" daughters. Women who tend to be perfectionistic, overachieving, and people-pleasing can develop this illness as part of their drive for acceptance.

Some athletic women, striving for success, equate being the thinnest with being the best athlete, particularly if their chosen sport emphasizes body-revealing clothing or light weight categories.

Winnie had always loved sports and her lifestyle revolved around working out. In high school, she was one of the few girls who used the weight room. She played field hockey and co-recreactional soccer, and she taught aerobics to help pay her way through college. After getting her degree in sports management, she was offered a job and moved to the East Coast. One of the first things she did was join a gym, where she worked out four or five times a week, taking aerobics classes and lifting weights. She was 23 and ready for a serious relationship. Her parents had divorced when she was 15, and she had never had a dating relationship longer than three or four months. She thought that to fit into "East Coast sophistication" and meet Mr. Right, she needed to lose a few pounds. She had always watched her weight, but now she wanted to be as thin as the women modeling workout clothes in her favorite magazines. She started a serious diet, eating only 800 calories a day. It was typical for her to check herself in the mirror several times a day and to weigh herself daily. She soon lost five pounds, and everyone told her how great she looked. She felt she still had a long way to go. She felt she had more energy than ever, and she felt lighter and more agile in her aerobics classes.

Winnie continued to diet and exercise and lost 20 pounds in four months. She found it easy to meet men at the gym or through parties and was dating two guys. She kept losing weight over the summer but felt she still looked fat in her aerobics leotard. At 5'6" she weighed 110 pounds and wanted to get down to 105. Her menstrual periods stopped, and once or twice she went in for pregnancy tests, fearing she had gotten pregnant. She also noticed that some of her hair was falling out and her skin was dry. By the fall, she was feeling tired and did not always get to work on time. She added a few more aerobics classes, thinking she needed to work out more to get back that great feeling of added energy she had had in the spring.

Winnie's work performance evaluation went poorly at mid-year. Her supervisor said she was often late for work and seemed to lack some of the ambition and drive needed in her job. Her life revolved around strict dieting, calorie counting, working out, and weighing herself every day. If she lost weight she felt great. If she did not, she felt depressed all day and was miserable to be around. She did not like going out with friends or dating, because she felt all these social activities involved fattening food or alcohol. She broke up with the guys she was dating and withdrew from most work and family activities. The only time she felt good was when she could fit into a size four dress, having become thinner than she had ever been in her life.

Tammy was a promising ballerina in her home town. She won a scholarship for a summer program at a national ballet company and went out of state for the whole summer to dance with them. She went on a drastic diet to lose weight before joining this program. During her first rehearsal, the ballet master told her she would never make it unless she lost 15 pounds. Tammy had already lost 5 pounds. She was desperate to lose more, but she was already living on carrots and rice cakes. She decided to stop eating every other day and ration her carrots to just five for breakfast and ten for dinner. She found she just couldn't drop much more weight and she felt fatter than all of the other dancers. Another ballerina told her to try smoking cigarettes and chewing gum. By midsummer, she was 7 pounds thinner, had a chronic cough, and found all she could think about was losing the remaining 8 pounds so that she could make it in the elite ballet company. When her parents visited the ballet company to see a performance, they were alarmed at her weight loss and smoking. They insisted she see a nutritionist and get off the cigarettes. She refused and got into shouting matches with her father and mother.

Winnie and Tammy are young women in the grip of anorexia nervosa. People with anorexia are characterized by their efforts to be in control— control of their bodies, their food intake, and their weight. The stories of entertainer Karen Carpenter (who died from medical complications of anorexia) and U.S. gymnast Christy Henrich (a member of the 1989 USA gymnastics team who died in 1994 from anorexia and bulimia) exemplify the serious and potentially fatal nature of this disorder.

Once an active woman has an established eating disorder—anorexia or bulimia (chapter 4)—she is on the road to the full syndrome of the female athlete triad. She is energy deprived. She is not her best in school, work, athletics, or personal relationships. She is too thin to win. However, by recognizing that her quest for thinness is damaging her body, she can begin to turn herself around and get the help she needs.

WHAT IS ANOREXIA?

Winnie and Tammy are intelligent, motivated women who obsessed about being fat and took dieting to the extreme. Anorexia is derived from the Greek word for lack of appetite. But the disorder is more complex and psychologically driven than simple appetite control. In addition to disordered eating, a person with anorexia has a serious disturbance in her body image and often experiences difficulty in her relations with other people. She doesn't recognize that she is extremely thin because she still perceives herself as fat and will never believe she is thin enough. No amount of persuasion by caring friends, family, or professionals can get her to change her distorted body image (see chapter 1 for a discussion of body image). But realize that this is not a voluntary or conscious denial of the truth. She truly feels fat and perceives herself as overweight. Her entire self-worth is connected to being thinner than anyone else. Her drive for extreme thinness is more than just the common desire to lose five or ten pounds, although it often begins with this idea.

There is often a very fine line between disordered eating behaviors and the eating disorder of anorexia. Whereas disordered eating is the occasional use of ineffective weight control measures, to be medically defined as anorectic a woman must meet all of the strict criteria outlined by the American Psychiatric Association (see list on page 70). When a woman has reached this clinical definition, she is dealing with a serious and life-threatening problem.

In the beginning stages of weight loss, many women report feeling great. Athletes may find that their performance improves for a time. This initial euphoria is partly due to the adrenaline rush that accompanies starvation. Your body is inspiring you to go hunting for more food by releasing adrenaline hormones. With some weight loss, a woman feels lighter and faster and may find some of her exercise is easier. That initial improvement is very transitory, because eventually anorexia takes away the fuel, muscles, and essential nutrients needed for physical activity. Any initial athletic performance improvement could also be from her increased dedication to exercise.

As she first loses weight, a woman may be rewarded with positive comments from her family, friends, and coaches about her looks and improved performance or accomplishments; comments such as, "You look great, have you lost weight?" or, "Losing that weight over the summer has really paid off in your mile-time." These comments then reinforce her belief in the advantages of losing more weight, and she becomes fixated on controlling her diet and appearance and on weighing herself (much like Winnie's experience at the beginning of this chapter). However, even in the early stages of anorexia, the starvation is harming vital organs like the heart and muscles and is impairing the brain's ability to think and concentrate. These changes are often subtle and may not be noticed by people close to her. Eventually, something gives, such as Winnie not doing well on her job evaluation or withdrawing from her friends. For an athletic woman, the first sign of anorexia may be that her athletic performance stops improving and she has to struggle harder to do what used to be easy and enjoyable. When your body does not have enough nutrition and reserves, as happens with anorexia, it runs out of fuel and has to slow down or stop.

When she starts to receive any negative comments about being too thin, a woman who has anorexia will often cover up her thin extremities with long sleeves, baggy pants, and dresses. It's not long before the energy deprivation and resulting loss of muscle eventually begin to hinder her athletic and mental abilities. Both Winnie and Tammy suffered from performance problems that were noticed by others but not recognized by themselves. This kind of denial is common in anorexia and is one of the reasons it is so difficult to treat.

Tammy continued to diet and dance. She was partnered with a male dancer for an upcoming performance. He told her that she was one of the heavier women he had worked with and she was even more determined to lose weight. Before their next practice together, she did not eat for two days and had lost a pound. However, she was not precise in her turns and could not stay en pointe for one of her solos. She missed a cue and her partner walked off stage disgusted. Tammy felt terrible about not dancing well and also felt lightheaded and had a headache. She had chronic pain in her lower legs and began taking large amounts of ibuprofen to make it through the day. She came earlier to practice and stayed later than everyone else, but still could not keep up with her new partner or seem to please him. Every practice ended with her in tears and pain.

A person with anorexia's drive for thinness and control becomes an overwhelming obsession. To achieve it, she tailors every aspect of her life to fulfill her weight goals—at the expense of her health—and is in danger of starving herself to death. She faces many other medical and psychological problems along the way. If you are around a woman with anorexia you may notice that she uses food-related rituals such as strict calorie counting, exercising to work off any calories consumed, and pushing food around her plate without eating it. She may prepare food for others but not have any herself. She may become defiant and secretive about her eating behavior and reject comments from people concerned about her health. She may take her underlying fears, insecurities, and conflicts and displace them into extreme concern about weight and eating, which she feels she can control to some degree.

From these descriptions, you may recognize anorexia in someone you know or even in yourself. Although disordered eating behaviors are red flags for eating disorders, clinicians can only officially diagnoses someone as having anorexia nervosa if the following four criteria are met:

1. Refusal to maintain body weight even though 15 percent or more below weight range expected for age and height
2. Intense fear of gaining weight
3. Body image distortion; feeling fat even when very underweight
4. Absence of three or more consecutive menstrual periods

Adapted, with permission, from the *Diagnostic and Statistical Manual of Mental Disorders*, Fourth Edition. Copyright © 1994 American Psychiatric Association.

The keys to the diagnosis and to understanding the psychological disturbance are the person with anorexia's fear of gaining weight and her perception of herself as fat even though she is very thin. Also important in the diagnosis is amenorrhea—a lack of menstrual periods for three months or more. Why do the menstrual periods stop? The lack of calories leads directly to a severe energy deficiency. The body is unable to meet its basic needs and cannot do certain functions. The first body function to shut down is that of reproduction. Menstrual cycles stop as the starving body tries to conserve energy.

There are two recognized subtypes of anorexia, restrictive anorexia and binge-purge anorexia. The restrictive type—in which the amount and type of food eaten is severely restricted—is the most common type. Binge-purge anorexia, on the other hand, is characterized by taking in a quantity of food (which may be considered a binge) and then using a method such as vomiting or taking laxatives to attempt to get rid of it. Binge-purge anorexia differs from bulimia in that the person who has it severely restricts her overall intake of calories. People with anorexia can alternate between both types of behaviors, but what is consistent is their marked body image distortion.

Winnie was unaware that her life had become restricted and revolved around her workouts and weighing herself. She did not realize that her work was suffering and that people were talking behind her back about how thin she was. She believed she was close to success because she could wear a size four, and she wanted to lose just a few more pounds. In reality, she was in danger of losing her job. Her supervisor was alarmed by her appearance and weight loss (almost 30 pounds in less than six months). She was no longer the enthusiastic, attractive woman hired right out of college. Instead she was thin, and forlorn looking; she appeared tired and exhausted. Her thin hair, dry skin, and the circles under her eyes made her look older than her age. She was not pursuing clients aggressively enough and had lost business for her firm. Her supervisor was worried that Winnie had a serious medical condition and took her aside one day to express her concerns. But Winnie told her that she was feeling great and working out. Privately, Winnie thought her boss was jealous of how great she looked since she had lost weight.

WHAT CAUSES ANOREXIA?

We wish we knew the causes! They are still under study and speculation. Cases of anorexia have been recorded since the late 1600s; it was a rare but recognized illness. However, many more cases have been recorded in the past 20 years. As we reviewed in chapter 1, a generation of women have been indoctrinated with the message that to be thin is to be happy and successful. Some athletes and active women falsely equate success or excellence in their sport with being thin (neglecting to consider their overall health). We all receive these messages, and some of us take them to the extremes of dieting and strict self-control. Women most likely to be affected are in the middle to high socioeconomic classes, are between the ages of 13 and 35, and come from developed societies around the world. There may be a genetic predisposition as well; studies show that identical twins are more likely to both have anorexia than nonidentical twins.

Theories about the causes of anorexia have ranged from it being a neurological disorder to a personality disorder to a psychiatric illness. For the woman with anorexia, striving for weight loss, obsessing about her weight, and dieting become automatic behaviors, behaviors she simply cannot stop even if she wants to. People who have anorexia are often experiencing a profound struggle between their bodies, their psyches, their families, and their cultures. Tammy's attempts to meet the conflicting demands of the ballet world, her body's need for nourishment, and the demands of her family are an example of this physical and psychological struggle. Winnie also had a conflict raging that was taking its toll on her health.

Symptoms of weight loss and body image distortion need to be seen as a cry for help, a smoke alarm going off to signal the fire of underlying psychological issues and problems. To understand and help someone recover, the causes of the fire—the person's distress—need to be addressed in professional treatment. In most cases, people who have anorexia do not recognize their emotional issues and are in deep denial about their weight loss and medical problems. Breaking through the denial is difficult. Part of treatment involves recognizing the underlying pain and problems, and working to treat these issues, as well as working on improved nutrition, energy intake, body image, and weight gain (see chapter 7).

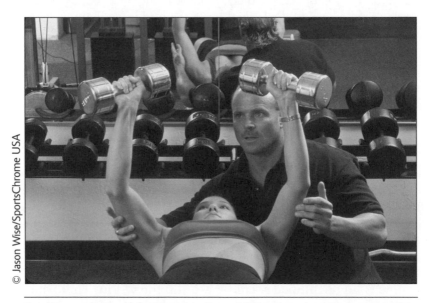

© Jason Wise/SportsChrome USA

Focusing on positive, strength-enhancing activities to lose or maintain your weight rather than restrictive diets is one way to ensure that you stay too fit to quit.

WHO IS AT RISK?

Accurate figures on anorexia have been kept only for the past few years. Most of the cases have been described in adolescent girls. In 1994, the American Psychiatric Association reported that 1 to 2 percent of young American girls fit the strict psychiatric definition. There are currently no statistics available on the estimated number of people with disordered eating behaviors that develop into anorexia. Today, as many as 1 in 250 adolescent girls in countries all over the world may be affected. Over 95 percent of cases occur in women, but men can also develop anorexia. Anorexia usually begins during adolescence but can occur as late as the early 30s. There are no statistics available to indicate whether active women are more or less at risk than nonexercisers.

Anorexia is not like the flu; it doesn't come and go quickly. Rather, it is a chronic illness that can take a long time to treat and is one of the most serious of young adult illnesses. People who have had anorexia report that even after years of treatment, they still have "anorectic thinking" and have to guard against a recurrence.

RECOGNIZING ANOREXIA

The earlier anorexia (or any eating disorder) is recognized and treated, the better the chances a woman won't do permanent damage to her heart, brain, bones, and kidneys. In long-term follow-up studies on people with anorexia, mortality rates are between 5 and 18 percent; causes of death are suicide and heart or kidney problems. Early recognition and prompt treatment of anorexia can prevent these deaths. The shorter the period of time someone has had psychological aspects such as body distortion and depression, the better her chances for recovery. If a woman recognizes she has a problem and then refers herself for help, she is even more likely to improve than if others try to force her into treatment. Even better, if she gets help when she first recognizes that she is obsessed about her weight and may have disordered eating patterns—before they develop into a full-blown eating disorder—she will have a much better chance of improvement and recovery and she will do less harm to her body.

Recognizing a woman with anorexia is easier than recognizing a woman with bulimia, who may be a normal weight or slightly overweight. Women with anorexia are starving and they look ill—too thin to win. In the initial stages, it can be hard to tell if someone is naturally thin or has lost weight because of intense physical training.

But if someone comments on her appearance, a woman in the beginning stages of anorexia will tell you that she still feels fat or that she wants to lose more weight. She may be very competitive about her weight loss and may point out another person who is even thinner and say that she wants to look like her. If you see her close up, she has lost muscle, her hair is thin on her scalp, and there is fine baby hair on her legs and arms. The bones of her skeleton protrude. Some people with anorexia feel they are fat all over their bodies. Others feel that only certain body parts need to be thinner. They may weigh, measure, and view themselves frequently and obsessively. Their self-worth is closely linked to a low body weight and the ability to avoid food. Figure 3.1 illustrates these and other warning signs of anorexia.

In contrast, a naturally thin person will recognize that she is thin, and she may be open to gaining weight. An athletically thin girl knows she is lean, and if she is convinced that gaining weight or increasing her muscularity would improve her athletic performance, she will more than likely be willing to do so.

Warning Signs for Anorexia

- Dramatic loss of weight (up to 15 percent or more below expected weight range)
- Denial; feelings of being fat even when thin; obsession with weight, diet, and appearance
- Use of food rituals or avoidance of social situations involving food
- Obsession with exercise; hyperactivity
- Sensitivity to cold
- Use of layers of baggy clothing to disguise weight loss
- Fatigue (in later stages)
- Decline in work, school, or athletic performance
- Growth of baby-fine hair over face and body, called lanugo hair
- Yellow tint to skin, palms, and soles of feet (from high levels of carotene)
- Hair loss, dry hair, dry skin, brittle nails
- Loss of muscle mass and tone
- No menstrual periods (amenorrhea)
- Slow pulse at rest, light-headedness on standing up quickly
- Constipation

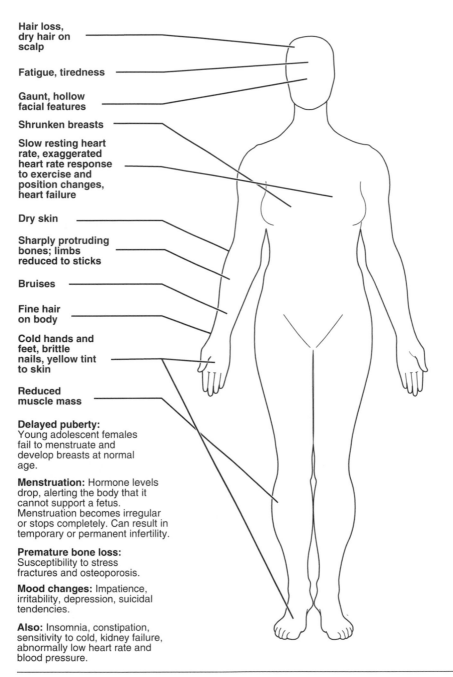

Hair loss, dry hair on scalp

Fatigue, tiredness

Gaunt, hollow facial features

Shrunken breasts

Slow resting heart rate, exaggerated heart rate response to exercise and position changes, heart failure

Dry skin

Sharply protruding bones; limbs reduced to sticks

Bruises

Fine hair on body

Cold hands and feet, brittle nails, yellow tint to skin

Reduced muscle mass

Delayed puberty: Young adolescent females fail to menstruate and develop breasts at normal age.

Menstruation: Hormone levels drop, alerting the body that it cannot support a fetus. Menstruation becomes irregular or stops completely. Can result in temporary or permanent infertility.

Premature bone loss: Susceptibility to stress fractures and osteoporosis.

Mood changes: Impatience, irritability, depression, suicidal tendencies.

Also: Insomnia, constipation, sensitivity to cold, kidney failure, abnormally low heart rate and blood pressure.

Figure 3.1 Effects of anorexia nervosa.

Reprinted, by permission, from B. Ludovise, 1992, "Eating disorders: Toll on the body," *Los Angeles Times,* December 6. Copyright © Los Angles Times Syndicate.

Winnie's boss recognized that something was going seriously wrong with Winnie. She noticed that Winnie had hair loss, dry skin, fatigue, extreme weight loss, and seemed to be obsessed with exercise and workouts at the gym. Yet even though she was extremely thin, Winnie continued to talk about losing weight. Her boss did not know that Winnie also had amenorrhea and constipation and often felt light-headed. When Winnie rebuffed her boss's initial effort to show concern, she knew she had to do something about Winnie's poor job performance. She called Winnie in for another meeting, and this time she concentrated on what was going wrong in the job. She pointed out Winnie's lateness and fatigue, her reluctance to take on extra clients, the client's complaints, and then contrasted those realities with Winnie's statement that nothing was wrong. She said that something had to improve and until it did Winnie was on probation. She suggested that Winnie get a medical checkup and join in more at the client parties. Winnie was shocked by her boss's warnings and was determined to show her boss that she could do better.

When **Tammy** went home after the summer session with the national ballet company, her parents were shocked at her appearance. She wore layers of baggy clothes and walked with a limp because of her leg pain. Her skin looked pale and slightly yellow. She seemed to have lost all of the muscle tone in her upper back and legs, and her ribs showed through her leotard. Tammy insisted that she felt fine and danced great. She told her parents she loved ballet and wanted to be a professional. She told them that everyone got lower-leg pain and that she really needed to lose more weight to make it in ballet. Her parents could not get through to her about the changes they noticed. Every family meal was a battle, with Tammy pushing food around and eating only a small amount of it. Tammy was in her senior year of high school and trying to balance school and ballet classes five nights a week. She slept only a few hours every night and looked tired all of the time.

In the beginning stages of the illness, a woman with anorexia may be energetic, happy, or overactive. She may report a euphoric feeling, with boundless energy during the initial stages of her weight loss. As you may remember from earlier in this chapter, this initial feeling of euphoria is due to the release of adrenaline. Only after significant body weight is lost do the signs of starvation develop. As subcutaneous fat is lost, she may often feel cold, have cold hands and feet, and dress in layers of clothes to both feel warm and disguise the weight loss.

She may grow a fine, baby type of hair, called lanugo hair, on her face, arms, and legs. Why? This hair is thought to be the body's attempt to keep warm. It is unique to and characteristic of anorexia. With decreased calorie intake, particularly a lack of protein and fat, women with this condition develop dry, brittle nails, dry hair, and patches of hair loss.

A woman with anorexia may be constipated and have low amounts of urine. A girl may not start her periods or her menstrual periods will stop, sometimes even before significant weight loss occurs. The reasons are not known. As semistarvation continues, there is a decline in mental and physical performance. For example, a top A student suddenly is struggling to get C's. In Winnie's case, she got a poor work evaluation and lost interest in dating. Blood sugar is low and fuel is lacking for both the brain and the body's muscles. Fatigue, loss of concentration, and lack of interest in usual activities is common.

Four to eight months after the onset of weight loss, work, academic, and athletic performance declines. Since many people who have anorexia are concerned with perfect performance, this decline is one way to help them recognize the toll their starvation is taking on their bodies and their lives. In later stages, medical problems develop as her body is forced to digest itself. The body breaks down muscles from the limbs and heart to obtain the protein needed for new cell growth each day. This muscle breakdown is dangerous to the heart and can lead to slow pulse, irregular heartbeats, and other problems.

Medical Problems

People with anorexia develop a characteristic yellow tinge to their skin, particularly noticeable on the palms and soles of the feet. It does not appear in the whites of their eyes. This yellow tint is caused by an elevated level of a substance called carotene. The increase in carotene is due to an alteration in the synthesis of vitamin A by the liver and is unique to anorexia. The body begins breaking down muscle, which can overload the kidneys. Kidney function is normal in the early stages of anorexia, but in later stages kidney function declines and can fail. Electrolytes, liver function, and calcium, phosphorus, and magnesium levels can also be abnormal in anorexia.

People with anorexia can develop a variety of heart problems. At first they may just have a slow pulse and low blood pressure. The slow pulse is sometimes confused with the low resting pulse of an athlete. The low resting pulse in someone with anorexia is caused by the slowdown of her metabolic processes because of starvation. Her pulse will rise with minimal exertion and with changes in position. The athlete, on the other hand, has a slow pulse due to the efficiency of her trained heart, which does not have to beat as fast in order to pump blood. The athlete will not have such an elevation in her pulse with minimal exertion. The athlete with anorexia will have the slow resting pulse of an athlete and the exaggerated increased heart rate response to exercise of someone with anorexia. The person with anorexia's blood pressure may fall dramatically when she stands up from a lying position. She is likely to feel dizzy and light-headed or even to pass out with sudden changes in position. In later stages of the illness, heart failure can occur as the body digests more of the heart muscle during starvation. Death has been reported from irregular heartbeats, heart failure, and seizures.

> Around Thanksgiving, headlines appeared in **Tammy's** local newspaper about the death of a young ballerina from another company, presumably from anorexia. Tammy and her family had known this young girl from ballet classes she and Tammy had taken together. Tammy was very upset at the death of her friend and went to the memorial service. Tammy understood what her friend must have been going through, starving herself to be a ballerina. She knew only too well the pressure to not eat and the pain and sense of failure of not being thin enough.

The body has a remarkable ability to sustain itself through the starvation of anorexia. Until 35 to 45 percent of body weight is lost, there may be no changes in any blood tests. All of the hormones of the female reproductive system are low, including estrogen, the hormone thought to be most important in keeping bones strong. The lack of estrogen is the principal reason these women have a pronounced loss of bone density that eventually leads to osteoporosis (see chapter 6). The osteoporosis may first be diagnosed after the occurrence of a serious

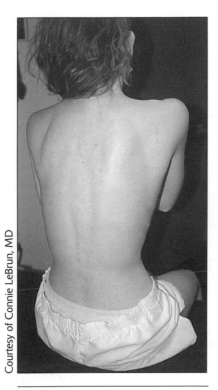

Courtesy of Connie LeBrun, MD

Figure 3.2 A patient with anorexia.

fracture. Many types of serious fractures have been reported in patients with anorexia, including crush fractures of the spine—wedge-shaped fractures resulting in a permanently bent spine just like the dowager's hump sometimes seen in postmenopausal women—stress fractures, and complete fractures, particularly in the hip or femur (the long bone of the upper leg). There is clear evidence from follow-up studies that the amount of bone mineral lost during anorexia is irreplaceable. The sooner osteoporosis is diagnosed and treated, the less serious it will be. The dietary inadequacies of anorexia can cause anemia, a low red-blood-cell count. Because of the low levels of red blood cells, the body has less oxygen-carrying capacity, which is certainly harmful to an athletic woman.

Women with anorexia do not look well. They look like starved, chronically ill patients. They lack a gleam in their eyes, a sheen in their hair, and their skin and nails appear dull and lifeless. When undressed, they appear skeletal (figure 3.2), yet they will look at themselves in the mirror and think they look fat, or at least not thin enough.

Winnie decided that the best way to improve her job performance was to work out more and get stronger. She tried going to a client party, but she felt like she did not fit in with the crowd that was drinking and eating. She resolved to get to work on time and made it in early for a week. After work she always went to the gym, usually after not eating anything all day. One evening she was running on the treadmill when she felt faint. She was barely able to get off the machine before passing out and collapsing on the floor. One of the personal trainers who had been watching her and had worked with her occasionally called 911. By the time the ambulance arrived, she had recovered consciousness but was still woozy. The

(continued)

paramedics took her to the emergency room, where she was evaluated and found to be dehydrated and severely underweight. The doctor gave her intravenous fluids and referred her to a specialist who treated eating disorders. The specialist was able to convince Winnie to see a psychologist and a nutritionist, as well as to get her parents involved. Winnie began a long and difficult road to recovery.

Psychological Problems

Many psychological issues underlie the starvation of anorexia. Remember how we referred to the symptoms as a smoke alarm, the warning that a fire—the fire of psychological conflict—is burning somewhere? The typical psychological profile of a woman with anorexia often reveals someone who turns to dieting and weight control to manage the chaos in her life. She is driven to be perfect in many ways and usually is a high achiever and hard worker. She may appear perfect on the outside, but she struggles with many identity and communication issues. These struggles can be part of the rite of passage through adolescence into adulthood. A woman with anorexia concentrates on her weight and appearance instead of dealing with these issues.

Anorexia is very much about being in control of food, of feelings, and of one's body. Feeling organized, disciplined, and at the center of attention become important parts of a woman with anorexia's life. Her sense of self-worth is likely to come from her ability to lose weight and remain in control and thin. She can never be thin enough, and the dieting disorder takes over her life.

However, many women who have anorexia escape detection because they are very good at denying their food restriction and at covering up. One patient told me that she was "good at PR," meaning that whenever someone tried to confront her with her extreme thinness, she always had an explanation and could charm the person into not prying further. The denial and intelligence of many women with this condition makes it very difficult for concerned friends and family to convince them get the medical and psychological help they need. We provide some ideas for getting a person into treatment in chapter 7; often it takes a serious medical problem for the woman with anorexia to go for help.

People with anorexia can be perfectionistic and maybe obsessive-compulsive and may be in denial that they have a problem. However, there comes a time when the self-control breaks down and they find themselves "overeating"—a "binge" that would be normal eating to most other people but that seems to them to be a huge transgression. It may have been due to physiological hunger or stress, but in some cases it may cause someone with anorexia to enter a cycle of bingeing and purging similar to seen in bulimia.

Women dealing with anorexia are often depressed. They have tied their self-worth to their appearance, and feel they can never be thin enough. They are at high risk for serious depression and even suicide. Even if a woman gets treatment and regains weight, the anorectic thinking can stay with her for years.

OVERCOMING ANOREXIA

Given the serious nature of anorexia, it is critical that we do all we can to prevent, recognize, and treat women before serious problems develop. Chapters 7 and 8 discuss treatment and prevention of anorexia and the female athlete triad disorders with which it is linked. If after reading this chapter you recognize yourself or someone you know as having anorexia, get into a treatment plan now. It can save your life.

After the memorial service for her ballerina friend, **Tammy's** mom could see she was really shaken. She took this time to talk to Tammy about what had been going on. Tammy broke down and told her mom that she knew what had happened to her friend—about all the pressure to not eat and to dance all day even if she was in pain. Something clicked inside Tammy, and she vowed this would not happen to her. She realized she loved to dance and if she could not make it as a ballerina, she would dance modern or with a company that didn't demand such perfection and thinness. She agreed to go to a doctor for a checkup. She started reading about anorexia and wrote a paper for her high school health class about it. But Tammy still found that thoughts of dieting, of being fat, or of being miraculously taller and thinner and a prima ballerina occupied her every waking thought. She found it nearly impossible to stop her very restrictive eating pattern.

Her family and doctor finally convinced her to get psychological treatment. After working six months with a treatment team made up of her family doctor, a psychologist, and a nutritionist, Tammy had gained a few pounds and could eat

(continued)

with the family without a huge fight. She had added some protein and milk to what she allowed herself to eat and felt that she had a bit more energy. She still had desires to be thinner but found she could talk about them with her therapist and family. Tammy found that it was a real struggle to eat with other people. She often sorted food into "forbidden" and "safe" groups. For so long she had denied herself anything with fat in it, or any chocolate, that these foods seemed like enemies. She had to work with the nutritionist for "permission" to eat these formerly forbidden foods. At times she would find herself automatically saying no to dessert or reaching for "fat-free" muffins. When she talked to friends about ballet, she again felt the urges to not eat and to be very thin and light so that she could float on the stage. She had many ups and downs as she worked with her treatment team on these issues. Whenever she felt hopeless, she wrote in a journal and shared some of it with her psychologist. She decided to stop ballet during her treatment and found she had more time for and interest in school, friends, and family activities. She and her family went to family therapy and became closer than they had been in years.

WHAT WINNIE'S AND TAMMY'S EXPERIENCES TEACH US

While Winnie was 23 years old and starting her first job, Tammy was 16 and took a scholarship for a summer dance program away from home. As they both faced different times of change, they responded to their different problems in a similar manner.

Using extreme exercise and dieting to handle transitions and pressure

Both women mistakenly turned to extreme exercise and dieting as a way of handling transitions and pressure in an attempt to be perfect. Tammy's pressure came from a ballet instructor who demanded she reach an impossible weight goal. Winnie pressured herself to lose weight as a way of fitting into a competitive work environment and meeting "Mr. Right." Both lost balance in their lives, turning to exercise and dieting and becoming self-preoccupied to such a degree that they were unable to see themselves objectively.

Action to take: When faced with times of transition, keep in touch with those friends and family who love you. If you are lonely or feel out of your element, express these feelings and get help and support. Realize that no one is perfect. If feelings of inadequacy overwhelm you, seek help from a counselor or psychologist. Don't try to control your feelings with diet and exercise.

Feeling fat in a thin body

Winnie and Tammy developed a distorted body image, feeling fat even when they were actually thin.

Action to take: If your diet leads you to being thinner than you have ever been in your life, yet you still think you are overweight, seek the advice and opinion of an expert in nutrition, psychology, or medicine. You have the characteristic thinking and body image distortion of someone who has anorexia. GET HELP!

Avoiding people who care

Both women isolated themselves from friends, family, and coworkers.

Action to take: If you find yourself doing this, ask yourself why. If it's because people who care about you are pointing out your extreme weight loss or unhealthy appearance and you don't want to hear it, then you are in denial of your serious problems. Maintain contact with your friends and family. Isolating yourself can lead to depression and further anorectic behavior and medical problems.

Ignoring absence of menses

Winnie and Tammy stopped having menstrual periods and did not realize this was a warning sign for which they should have sought medical care.

Action to take: If your periods stop for three months or more, get a medical evaluation. The cessation of menstrual periods (amenorrhea) is a warning sign of anorexia, as well as bone loss and increased chance of stress fracture (see chapter 5).

Dismissing the concerns of others

Both women ignored concerns and attempts to intervene from family, friends, and coworkers.

Action to take: Listen to those who care about you. They recognize that you are struggling, even though you insist everything is fine. You may be strictly controlling your diet and exercise, while ignoring underlying emotional conflicts. Everyone faces problems as we go through life, but denying problems does not solve them. Seek professional help.

Ignoring symptoms of medical problems

They developed and attempted to ignore medical problems, such as injuries that didn't heal and fainting. Winnie passed out while running on a treadmill and was taken to the hospital. Tammy tried to dance through leg pain, ending every practice in tears.

Action to take: People with anorexia have such a strong sense of control and denial, they are likely to not recognize serious underlying medical problems. If you take pain medication daily, pass out, or have injuries that do not heal, discuss these problems with your coach, trainer or a medical professional. Reconnect with your body and what it is telling you. Recognize that you need help to make adjustments in your training and diet to deal with these issues.

What Winnie and Tammy Did Right

- ◆ Entered treatment before developing irreversible physical and mental changes
- ◆ Reconnected with family and friends
- ◆ Expressed their feelings through writing and speaking
- ◆ Began eating more nutritious foods
- ◆ Continued working with their treatment teams

If anorexia is treated in its early stage by a combination of medical, nutritional, and psychological help, permanent damage to the body and mind can be avoided. Voluntarily going for help is a good indication you will recover. See chapter 7 for more information on getting treatment.

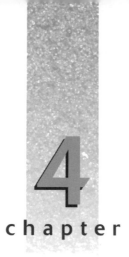

chapter

Out of the Kitchen
and Into the Closet:
Bulimia Nervosa

Do you or your friends or relatives worry about weight? Have you been tempted to use purging techniques, or do you know people who have? We are all bombarded with pressure about our weight, and if we are athletic or active women, this pressure might influence how we think our weight affects our success in sport. However, we also are learning that the best way to stay healthy and avoid the female athlete triad is to fuel our bodies with the energy and nutrients they need—not to diet, or starve, or purge. Getting the right information about nutrition, having a positive body image, and maintaining appropriate body weight will keep us performing at our best.

Still, faced with pressure to lose weight, we know that some women turn to disordered eating practices such as those described in chapter 2. Many active women use purging techniques to get rid of food (and guilt) after eating in a misinformed effort to lose weight. There are some women who erroneously believe that they can lose weight (and thus be successful and happy) by adopting these bulimic behaviors. This chapter defines bulimia, describes how it damages the body, and explains who is at risk.

Jessica was a college swimmer who had dreamed of making the U.S. Olympic swim team since she was 10 years old. However, she quit the sport she loved in her junior year of college. Her parents and teammates were shocked that she retired before her last chance to qualify. She told them that she had outgrown the sport, was bored, and wanted to get more out of college. She said she wanted to date and take late-morning classes so she could sleep in.

Her roommate, however, knew that Jessica had been battling bulimia for two years and was starving herself all day, then bingeing and throwing up at night. In an effort to improve her swimming times, Jessica went on a drastic diet to lose weight her freshman year. Her strict diet often left her famished by the

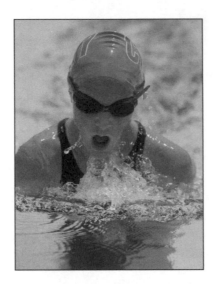

evening, and she found herself eating several bowls of cereal and "blowing her diet." She felt like a failure at losing weight. One night after bingeing on cereal, she discovered how to make herself vomit. Her performance on the swim team got worse instead of better. Jessica had been feeling tired for months and was not making her times in swim practice. She fasted every morning, binged while she studied, and vomited at night when she thought her roommates were asleep. She did not think the vomiting would cause any serious problems, but when I first met Jessica she had come to the health center after vomiting blood for four days in a row and feeling light-headed. She told me that she was really frightened and had decided to quit the swim team. "I was just so tired of all the weigh-ins and of

> being hungry all the time and having to vomit or use laxatives to keep my weight down. It wasn't worth it to me anymore."

Bulimia is one of several serious eating disorders that is part of the female athlete triad. People with bulimia may not appear to be too thin to win, but the medical and psychological problems they experience impair physical and mental performance.

WHAT IS BULIMIA?

Bulimia nervosa, from the Greek word for ox hunger, is a complicated disorder characterized by repetitive cycles of dieting, then overeating—bingeing—followed by behaviors that get rid of, or purge, the food eaten. A woman with bulimia may feel that her life is an unpredictable roller-coaster ride. One moment she is safely strapped in, moving along slowly. Then begins an invigorating and anxious upward ride to the top, a moment of pause as tension builds, then a terrifying plunge down to the depths. After the thrill of the ride, she wants to do it again. People who have bulimia face great shifts in weight, body image, and mood, and may seem to be addicted to this out-of-control behavior.

Whereas anorexia is characterized by strict control of food intake, bulimia is a loss of control. The affected person plunges into recurrent episodes of dieting or restricting food intake. This restriction then leads to uncontrollable hunger resulting in automatic or unconscious overeating (see p. 44, chapter 2). The person with bulimia feels guilty and ashamed that she has blown her diet; she feels like a failure. She may turn to purging—not just to get rid of food but also to get rid of bad feelings and emotions. Purging may bring her a sense of relief and a resolution to the stress and guilt of overeating. This sense of relief completes the cycle. The relief is the hook that makes bulimia such an addictive behavior. The cycle repeats itself the next day; she resolves to diet, then inadvertently overeats again. The cyclic nature of the bingeing and purging is eventually experienced as a compulsion and need. In this way it mimics other addictive behaviors such as alcohol or drug abuse and is incredibly difficult to stop.

Understanding the cycle of bulimia requires understanding the physiological effects of semistarvation (see page 41, chapter 2). Anytime you restrict your food intake, as when dieting and fasting, your body reacts to its lack of nourishment by releasing hunger hormones that command your body to eat. Therefore, dieting and fasting inevitably lead to hunger and overeating (see figure 4.1). You may use caffeine, appetite suppressants, decongestants like Sudafed, or even diet pills to suppress the hunger. However, once the hunger hormones finally take over, you will want to overeat to compensate. For someone with bulimia, though, the guilt of overeating and failing the diet leads to anxiety and self-loathing, which lead to a compulsion to get rid of the calories just consumed.

Jessica never ate before swim practice and drank Diet Coke to give her energy to get through her morning classes. She allowed herself only one bagel before her afternoon workout. If she felt hungry for more, she drank another Diet Coke or took a Dexatrim diet pill. At dinner she tried to eat only salad. The downside to her strict diet was that by eight or nine o'clock, while studying, she would eat two to five bowls of cereal. Afterward, she felt bloated, gross, and disgusted with herself, and she secretly vomited in the bathroom. Vomiting made her feel light-headed, but she felt a great sense of relief at getting rid of the food. She was embarrassed to be doing this but found it became an almost daily pattern that she had to hide from her roommates.

People with bulimia may purge by using one or more of several different methods including taking diuretics, laxatives, or enemas; forcing themselves to vomit; or exercising excessively (and obsessively) in an effort to burn calories. In the strict clinical definition of bulimia, the binge eating and purging behaviors occur an average of at least twice a week for three months. However, a person may use bulimic behaviors occasionally but not be clinically diagnosed as having bulimia nervosa. Recognizing and preventing these behaviors is important in stopping them from developing into a full-blown eating disorder. See page 93 for a list of symptoms and signs of bulimic behavior.

Bulimia has been recognized and defined only recently. The American Psychiatric Association first published diagnostic criteria for bulimia in 1980 in its Diagnostic and Statistical Manual, and it revised these criteria in 1994. A key part of the definition is the compulsive and repetitive nature of the purging.

Diagnostic Criteria for Bulimia

1. Repeated episodes of binge eating, at least twice a week for three months
2. Feeling of lack of control during eating binges
3. Use of one or more purging methods: self-induced vomiting, laxatives, diuretics, or excessive exercise
4. Overconcern with body shape or weight

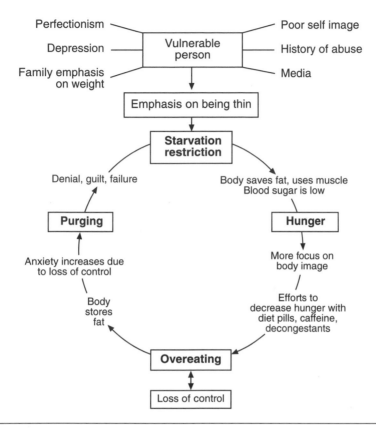

Figure 4.1 The cycle of bulimia.

But there is a problem with limiting the definition to such strict criteria. By the time a woman exhibits the symptoms in this strict definition, she may be in the throes of a very serious and potentially fatal condition that could have been avoided or treated if it had been caught earlier. You can recognize bulimic behaviors early and get help to break the cycle before you do too much damage to your body, your fitness, and your psyche.

In addition to the classic eating disorders anorexia nervosa and bulimia nervosa, the APA has defined another type of eating disorder. This disorder is described in both athletic and nonathletic women. It has a broader definition, which includes people who meet the criteria for anorexia but do not have amenorrhea (absence of menstrual periods), as well as those who binge eat without purging, and who chew and spit out food instead of swallowing it or purging. If you recognize that you (or a friend or teammate) meet one or more of the criteria listed, we urge you to seek professional help before your performance and health are harmed by the disordered eating.

Criteria for Eating Disorder Not Otherwise Specified

1. Meets all the criteria for anorexia nervosa (see page 70) but has regular menses

2. Meets all the criteria for anorexia nervosa except that despite significant weight loss, current weight is in the normal range

3. Meets all the criteria for bulimia nervosa except that purging behavior occurs less than twice a week for less than three months

4. Uses purging behavior after eating small amounts of food

5. Repeatedly chews and spits out, but does not swallow, food

6. Recurrent episodes of binge eating without the use of purging methods

Adapted, with permission, from *Diagnostic and Statistical Manual of Mental Disorders*, Fourth Edition. Copyright © 1994 American Psychiatric Association, p. 550.

WHO IS AT RISK?

When I ask my patients with bulimia how many other women they know with this problem, they give me different answers. Some think they are the only ones; others say that at least a third of their friends have similar troubles. Since bulimia is a hidden disorder, it may be difficult to find out how many women are suffering.

Many psychologists believe there is an epidemic of bulimia, perhaps because of our increasingly consumption-based society, in which the mixed message is, "You can have your cake and eat it too" and "You can never be too thin." This disorder was almost unknown 30 years ago. Now doctor's offices and psychologist's waiting rooms are filled with patients with bulimia, and the bathrooms of sororities and dormitories are filled with purging women. Accurate figures about how many people use bulimic techniques are really unknown. Using the strict psychiatric criteria, the APA estimates that between 1 and 4 percent of young women have this disorder. Some studies have found that up to 70 percent of gymnasts are at risk, and 20 percent meet the clinical definition (see page 88). About 90 percent of those who have bulimia are women, and 10 percent are men.

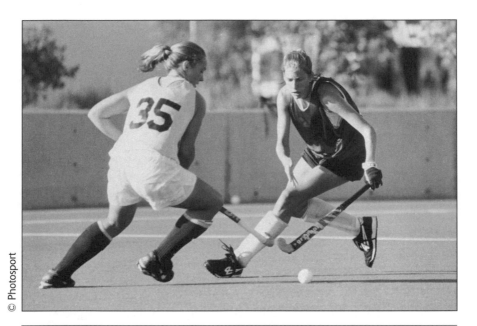

By understanding the risks of dieting and disordered eating practices and focusing on nourishing your body for your optimal performance, you can prevent yourself from falling into the triad trap.

Tracy gained 10 pounds her first year of college, but her roommate seemed to have no such problems. They were both on the field hockey team. Tracy seemed to eat just as much as her roommate, but she gained weight whereas her roommate didn't. One day after practice, Tracy's roommate told her that all she needed to do was to stick her finger down her throat and throw up whenever she thought she had eaten too much. Her roommate had been doing it since 10th grade and said, "It works for me." She said, "Lots of girls do it."

Some people may be more susceptible to developing bulimia, including chronic dieters with low self-esteem and negative body images. These people place high stakes on losing weight and base their self-worth on how successful they are at sticking to their diets. Often chronic dieters aim for an unachievable goal and then become depressed when they fail to reach it.

Women with a history of depression, impulse control disorders, or anxiety disorders, and those who have been victims of sexual abuse are also at greater risk. However, even women at high risk of developing bulimia can avoid it by recognizing dangerous dieting practices and taking preventive action.

> Although **Jessica** felt disgusted by her vomiting, she found she couldn't stop it. If she had a really good swim workout or did well on a test, she celebrated by eating more at dinner. Even though this was a reward for her performance, she still felt driven to throw up after the meal. If she didn't, she felt fat, guilty, and anxious. After she threw up, she felt relieved. The sense of relief that Jessica felt was the hook that kept her bingeing and purging.

RECOGNIZING BULIMIA

A woman with bulimia is not easily recognized. She can be normal weight or slightly overweight and almost any age, race, or educational background. Bulimia is a diverse disorder that includes many types of eating practices. Although people with bulimia have distorted body images and fears of getting fat, they are not as thin as people with anorexia. However, they constantly strive to be thinner, and their sense of self-worth is tied to how much they weigh.

> **Rosie** was a college gymnast who had extreme weight pressures. She had been a promising junior gymnast, headed for the Olympics, but she did not make the cut in the final tryouts. She accepted a college scholarship but did not seem to live up to her potential. She often fell off the balance beam in tough meets and thus tried to avoid competing on the beam. Rosie suffered from frequent sore throats. In her junior year, she had an episode of severe upper-abdominal pain and had to be hospitalized. During her hospitalization, she revealed that she had been using bulimic techniques for years to try to make the restrictive weight for gymnastics. Her sore throats were due to vomiting, and she was afraid of the beam because she often was light-headed and dizzy. No one had ever guessed that she had bulimia, not the doctors who treated her medical problems nor the coaches who had tried to get her to stick with the beam. Her teammates did not know that she vomited two to four times a day.

It can be hard to recognize bulimia, even in a roommate or close friend, because people who have it hide their behavior. They are ashamed of their overeating and subsequent vomiting or other form of purging. A woman with bulimia may eat a lot and then disappear to the bathroom, or she may hoard or even steal food and eat in secret. But, although a woman struggling with bulimia wants to keep her behavior secret, she can never completely hide. Her disorder can come to light accidentally, as when a roommate finds signs of her vomiting. The purging behavior can leave behind traces such as the odor of vomit on the breath or the following:

- ✦ Scabs or scars on knuckles. Vomiting by sticking a finger down one's throat can cause scabs and even scars on the backs of the knuckles, where the fingers have rubbed against the teeth.

- ✦ Swollen, persistently puffy face and cheeks. If the vomiting has been prolonged, the salivary glands (parotid glands) around the cheeks may become chronically swollen, giving the person with bulimia a chipmunk-cheek appearance that can persist for weeks and even months after she stops vomiting. Bulimia is the only disorder other than mumps that results in enlarged parotid glands. The swollen, "fat-face" appearance can be extremely distressing to the person who has bulimia and can cause her to redouble her efforts to lose weight.

- ✦ Broken blood vessels in face and eyes. If the vomiting is very forceful, blood vessels in the white part of the eyes, the nose, the mouth, and even the cheeks can burst.

- ✦ Sore throats and dental problems. Vomiting can lead to chronic sore throats, foul breath, dental cavities, and loss of tooth enamel.

- ✦ Abdominal symptoms. People with bulimia have a lot of abdominal symptoms even when they are not actually purging. Those who abuse laxatives experience episodes of abdominal bloating, diarrhea and constipation (when off the laxatives), abdominal pain that mimics appendicitis, ovarian cysts, or irritable bowel disease. Vomiting can bring acid from the stomach into contact with the esophagus, and symptoms of heartburn, acid reflux (also known as GERD—gastro-esophageal reflux disorder), and ulcers are common. In rare situations, the overeating can lead to rupture of the stomach, and the vomiting can cause tears and bleeding from the esophagus and stomach.

- ✦ Rapid weight changes. Most people with the disorder experience rapid fluctuations in weight. Their weight can change two to five pounds overnight because of dehydration. Some women gain a few pounds over several days from premenstrual water retention, but frequent changes of two to five pounds overnight are unheard of unless a person is dehydrating and then rehydrating through repetitive purging, use of laxatives or diuretics, and overeating. The weight loss is mostly due to loss of valuable body fluids and leads to a chronically dehydrated state. The person may feel thinner, but all that was lost is body water, seriously jeopardizing health and performance.

◆ Erratic performance. In addition to weight fluctuation, erratic performance in work, sport, and academics is a problem. Dehydrated is the worst way to be if you are athletic. Even 1 percent dehydration (a loss of one pound in a 100-pound person) impairs coordination, balance, and speed and slows reaction time. Think of how you feel at the end of a hot day when you have become dehydrated—you feel headachy, tired, light-headed, and thirsty. A woman with bulimia experiences these conditions frequently. Painful muscle cramps and soreness can result from dehydration and the loss of minerals that occur with purging. Bulimia can lead to low blood sugar, the fuel on which your brain depends. Low blood sugar can affect memory and concentration. Now imagine Rosie, the dehydrated gymnast, doing back flips on a four-inch-wide balance beam! Her chances for error were dramatically increased, and it is no wonder she feared this event.

◆ Irregular or absent menstrual periods. The energy drain caused by bulimia can result in amenorrhea (absence of menstrual periods) or infrequent or irregular periods. Menstrual problems like these indicate a lack of estrogen and other hormones that are essential for building strong bones—a situation that can lead to stress fractures and eventually to osteoporosis, another component of the female athlete triad.

A medical problem caused by purging can bring a person with bulimia to the doctor's office. Jessica sought help when she vomited blood. Rosie was hospitalized with frightening abdominal pain before her bulimia was detected, even though warning signs had been present for years. Others may seek help when they are fed up with having the eating disorder run their lives.

Sometimes women are discovered to have bulimia and are forced into treatment by friends, family, or coaches. One athlete I worked with was discovered vomiting by a teammate. She was the top gymnast on her team, but she had always fought weight issues. She had learned to vomit when she was 10 years old and had been doing it for seven years. Her teammate told the coach, and the coach immediately pulled her off the team and made her seek medical care. All the team members were put on notice that any evidence of these problems meant they would also be kicked off the team (and many of the other members of the team also had the disorder). Instead of helping these athletes get treatment, however, this threat drove them to be even more secretive about their behavior.

> **Rosie** came to see me in the clinic after her hospitalization. Like most people with bulimia, she denied that her physical problems were caused by her behavior. And like many athletes with bulimia, she did not realize that the disorder could harm her performance. She believed she still had a lot of weight to lose, even though she was thinner than most women and was at an acceptable weight for her sport. She had heard some horror stories about what bulimia could do to her body, and a few scary things had happened to her. She admitted to me that once after vomiting she had felt her heart racing and had been so dizzy that she had had to lie down. Her heart rate was more than 180 beats per minute, and she couldn't stand up for long without everything spinning. Despite these experiences, once she felt better, she forgot how scared she had been.

Bulimia is a serious medical illness with potentially lethal consequences such as heart irregularities, dehydration, and rupture of the stomach. Most people who have it do not want to hear about these consequences. Many of them have been vomiting for years, and because they are in denial they don't think that anything harmful has happened because of it. Most of my patients do not want a lecture, but they do need to know what can happen to them if they continue their purging. Sometimes learning about the risks of purging behavior can encourage someone to stop.

Some of the medical problems that result from bingeing and purging are temporary; others are permanent. Permanent, irreversible changes can include the loss of dental enamel, hiatal hernias, and osteoporosis. Depending on the type and frequency of purging behaviors used, common symptoms include dehydration, heart irregularities, muscle cramps, amenorrhea, and gastrointestinal problems (see figure 4.2, p. 97). Cardiac abnormalities are the most serious.

Does Purging Work?

Are you surprised to hear that purging does not effectively remove all of the food a person eats during a binge? Self-induced vomiting may only remove one-third to one-half of what has been eaten, because the body is designed to efficiently and quickly digest food. The stomach empties into the intestine 10 to 20 minutes after eating, and most of the calories from the food are absorbed there within a few minutes. Even vomiting immediately after eating does not prevent the body from absorbing some calories. Experienced practioners of bulimic behavior studied in laboratory settings could not fully empty their stomachs after a binge. Anywhere from 20 to 60 percent of swallowed food remained or had already moved to the small intestine, where the calories are quickly and efficiently absorbed.

Laxatives and diuretics only eliminate water and important electrolytes, not fat or calories. Thus, purging by using laxatives and diuretics leads to dangerous dehydration, not loss of body fat. Actually, repetitive purging and dehydration can, paradoxically, cause weight gain. The body does not like to be dehydrated from purging or any other cause. In response, the body produces a hormone called aldosterone, which causes the kidneys to retain water and electrolytes (e.g., sodium). When a person with bulimia temporarily stops purging and dehydrating, aldosterone causes the body to hold onto water. As a result, someone who does not purge for several days will become bloated and may gain two to five pounds in water weight overnight. She may feel like her body is suddenly fat and her hands and face are puffy. This is a very frightening feeling and can lead right back to purging.

The negative effects of purging, such as dehydration, electrolyte imbalance, and energy deficiency, are all more detrimental to performance—and more dangerous—than carrying a couple of extra pounds of body weight. In fact, those pounds might very well consist of the muscle you need to take your performance to greater heights.

It has been observed that women at risk for disordered eating have begun these behaviors after reading about them in a book or magazine or hearing about them from others. If after reading this book you feel any urge to begin these practices, run, don't walk, to the sections in chapters 2 and 3, and in this chapter, that discuss the serious medical and psychological problems that can develop. The intent of this book is to guide you to an improved body image and to effective weight control.

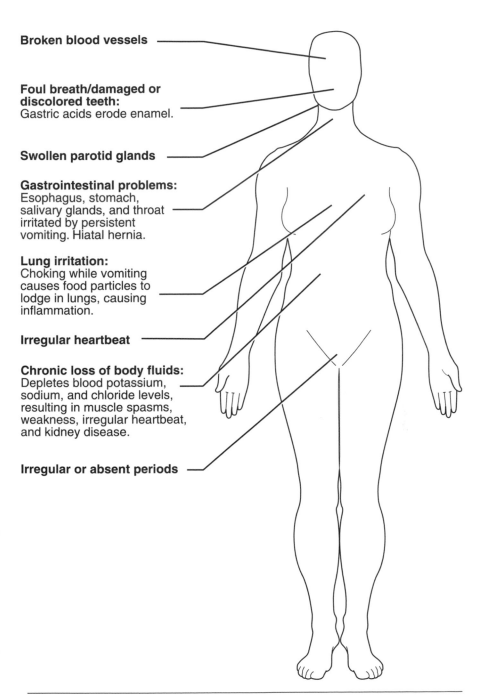

Broken blood vessels

Foul breath/damaged or discolored teeth:
Gastric acids erode enamel.

Swollen parotid glands

Gastrointestinal problems:
Esophagus, stomach, salivary glands, and throat irritated by persistent vomiting. Hiatal hernia.

Lung irritation:
Choking while vomiting causes food particles to lodge in lungs, causing inflammation.

Irregular heartbeat

Chronic loss of body fluids:
Depletes blood potassium, sodium, and chloride levels, resulting in muscle spasms, weakness, irregular heartbeat, and kidney disease.

Irregular or absent periods

Figure 4.2 Effects of bulimia nervosa.

Reprinted, by permission, from B. Ludovise, 1992, "Eating disorders: Toll on the body," *Los Angeles Times,* December 6. Copyright © Los Angles Times Syndicate.

Purging by Vomiting

Self-induced vomiting is the best known of the bulimic purging behaviors. A woman with bulimia may use her hand to activate the gag reflex in the back of her throat and vomit. She may use foul-tasting materials like mustard and salty water or a poison antidote called ipecac to reliably induce vomiting. Some people can just think about vomiting and do so.

Vomiting by any means results in losses of water, sodium (Na+), hydrogen (H+), potassium (K+), chloride (Cl−), and magnesium (Mg+). The sodium loss leads to further depletion of water and dehydration. The loss of hydrogen and chloride leads to a change in the delicate acid and base balance in the body, causing potential heart and muscle problems. The loss of potassium can cause irregular heartbeats and muscle cramps. The combination of changes can cause serious heartbeat irregularities.

Vomiting takes a toll on the psyche as well as on the body. It usually is practiced in solitude fairly soon after a meal. It is difficult for someone who has bulimia to vomit after group meals and keep it a secret. On college campuses, there are bathrooms known for privacy where students have told me that there is a line of people waiting to vomit. Vomiting can tear the esophagus or rupture the stomach. Either can be fatal if the acidic contents of the stomach are spread into the chest or abdominal cavities. Troubling, but less serious, are stomach ulcers and esophageal bleeding, hiatal hernias, and erosion of dental enamel. Cases of pneumonia have also been reported when people with the disorder accidentally inhale vomited material.

Ipecac—sold over the counter as an antidote to accidental poisoning—contains a chemical that induces vomiting within a few minutes after ingestion. Women who are too timid to use their hands or who cannot induce vomiting on their own may use ipecac sporadically or regularly. Frequent use of the chemical has been found to cause irreversible cardiac and skeletal muscle damage. Because of the serious and permanent damage ipecac causes, it should never be used as a purging agent. One of the things I insist that patients do is to toss out all bottles of ipecac at home or bring them in for disposal in the medical clinic.

At first **Jessica** found it hard to make herself vomit. She was not eating all day and was worried about making weigh-ins for the swim team. She felt so disgusted with herself for blowing her strict diet and eating three bowls of cereal that she was desperate to try anything. She had read in a magazine about women who made themselves vomit, and at first she thought it was a horrible thing to do. But alone, angry, and anxious to undo all her overeating, she tried sticking her finger down her throat. Afterward, she felt dizzy and tired, and she had a headache. As vomiting became a nightly habit, she found she always had a sore throat, puffy eyes, and looked and felt tired. Once after vomiting, she had burst blood vessels in her eye and had a bloody nose, which she had to explain to her roommates (she made up a story about blowing her nose really hard). She found it hard to get up in the mornings for early swim practice because she felt "washed out." She tried pushing it but could not get into fourth gear for a sprint. At least twice a week she had bad muscle cramps or charley horses in her calves or toes, usually while swimming. Later she learned that the vomiting was draining the potassium and sodium as well as some fluid from her body, leaving her dehydrated and prone to muscle cramps and slower times in the pool. Her diet was so unbalanced, what with the fasting, Diet Cokes, and nightly cereal binges, that she lacked protein to build muscle and adequate carbohydrate to refuel her muscles after swim practices. No wonder she felt tired and wasn't swimming well. She also was not getting any iron in her diet, so she was developing iron deficiency anemia and her blood had less oxygen-carrying capacity.

Abusing Laxatives

Various studies have found that laxatives are abused by anywhere from 18 to 75 percent of people who have bulimia. These laxatives are widely available over the counter. Most of them contain the chemicals cascara or phenophtalein. Phenophtalein was recently taken off the market because of concerns about serious side effects.

Laxative abuse associated with bulimia is marked by rituals and secretive use patterns. The abuser hides her behavior because of the shameful nature of having extreme amounts of diarrhea and the difficulty of explaining the practice to others. One patient of mine regularly bought laxatives at four different stores to avoid detection. Another carefully laid out the night's laxative tablets, counting them out according to how "good" or "bad" she had been that day. Some women use large doses of laxatives late at night when others in their households have gone to bed. They have painful cramps and profuse diarrhea during the remainder of the night, sometimes sleeping only for an hour at a time.

Does the embarrassment, pain, and expense of laxatives result in weight loss? Is it worth it to put yourself through the self-abusive practice of overdosing on laxatives? The answer is a clear no! The reason this practice is ineffective is that no laxative stops the body from absorbing any food or calories. Instead, it acts only on the large intestine, far down the digestive system, after all the calories and nutrients have been absorbed in the small intestine. A laxative increases the contractions of the muscle in the intestine. It empties the large intestine of undigested food and fiber and prevents the absorption of water. Many people with bulimia get "hooked" on laxatives because they feel lighter and as though they have lost weight after using them. In reality, laxative abuse does not result in loss of fat; what looks like weight loss is simply dehydration.

> **Rosie**, the gymnast, had tried using laxatives when she couldn't lose weight quickly enough. She started by taking one or two pills the night before a weigh-in. She had a really loose bowel movement the next morning. She felt lighter but did not lose much weight. Next she tried taking four pills at once, and she had really painful stomach cramps. Diarrhea started in two hours, and she was up all night going to the bathroom. After that she resolved not to use laxatives again, but she did not have a bowel movement for three days and felt really bloated. She felt so uncomfortable that she took four pills and again had painful diarrhea all night. She found she could not have a bowel movement without using laxatives, and soon she was using them nightly just to be regular. Many nights she took more than four pills, and she lost a lot of sleep as well as getting dehydrated. She often felt dizzy in gymnastics practices, and she hated doing the balance beam.

There is a high price to pay for abusing laxatives. They induce painful diarrhea, sometimes containing blood. They are likely to irritate the delicate lining of the intestine and can cause hemorrhoids, painful dilated veins around the rectum that can bleed. Laxatives force electrolytes like potassium and sodium as well as water from your body, putting you at risk for dehydration, cramps, and skipped heartbeats. If you use laxatives often, your body can become dependent on them to even have a bowel movement. They damage the nerve cells in the wall of the intestine, which leads to a paralyzed or "lazy" colon, or what physicians call a cathartic colon. If you have been taking large amounts of laxatives and suddenly stop taking them, you may experience colon paralysis and have no bowel movements for days.

Taking Appetite Suppressants

People who have bulimia often turn to appetite suppressants in an effort to stop eating. They may use caffeine for its mild appetite-suppressant effect. Caffeine is also a weak diuretic; it draws water out of the body and thus makes a person feel lighter. The downside of caffeine is that it can make you jittery, dehydrated, and hungry when its effect wears off. People with bulimia may also turn to decongestants to suppress their appetites. Decongestants are weak stimulants and mild appetite suppressants. Their side effects are irritability, increased heart rate, and dry mouth.

Stronger appetite suppressants, prescribed in waves of fads, claim to aid in losing body fat and make weight miraculously and rapidly disappear. But each fad has subsequently proven to have serious side effects and to provide no effective long-term weight loss. One recent appetite suppressant therapy, Fen-Phen, was used by millions until the serious side effect of heart valve malformations was reported. Before Fen-Phen was pulled off the market, millions of normal-weight women were using it to lose a few pounds.

As discussed in chapter 2, weight loss is rarely indicated for an athlete in training or competition. People are different, and there is no one optimal weight that all athletes in a given sport must attain in order to compete. An athlete is much better off concentrating on her training, strength, fitness, nutrition, and technique than on how much she weighs.

Abusing Diuretics

Diuretics are another over-the-counter or prescription medication abused by people with bulimia. The over-the-counter diuretics are directly marketed to women for symptomatic relief of "that bloated feeling." They are common ingredients in remedies for premenstrual syndrome. These compounds include medications like pamabrom or ammonium chloride that induce the kidneys to get rid of water in the body. These medications, especially those containing ammonium chloride, all cause dehydration and electrolyte and acid base disorders.

Some people with bulimia also use stronger, prescription diuretics. These are potent medications capable of removing one to five pounds of water from the body. They are very dangerous drugs, causing severe dehydration and electrolyte disturbances resulting in cardiac arrhythmia, skeletal muscle spasms, and fainting.

> **Eileen**, who had just turned 30, had had bulimia for eight years, but was doing well in therapy when I met her. I asked her how bulimia had changed her life. Her bulimia started during her senior year in college. She was on the tennis team and was losing many of her matches. After a particularly difficult loss to a player she should have beaten, she went on an eating binge of chocolate and ice cream. Horrified, she then forced herself to throw up. Strangely, she felt better after vomiting.
>
> Eileen said she felt caught in the cycle of starving during the day, then bingeing late at night and vomiting. She almost had a ritual for how she vomited, and she hid what she was doing from her friends and family. The bulimic practices became more important than school, work, her friends, or tennis. Two years after she started, she could not eat a regular meal of more than 400 calories without feeling anxious or needing to vomit. If she had a stressful day at work, she knew she could feel better by eating her favorite food and then throwing it up. Her work and her friendships suffered.
>
> Alarmed when she did not get a promotion at work, she became anxious and depressed. Unable to sleep, she went to see a physician to get a sleeping pill. Soon she was talking about her bulimia, and the physician helped her deal with the issues of stress, anxiety about her job, and difficult family relationships. She joined a therapy group for women with eating disorders and kept a journal. As she began to talk about the things that were bothering her, she found that she had less need to overeat and vomit. A year and a half after starting therapy, she had not thrown up in two months and was enjoying work and playing tennis again.

Exercising Excessively

Recently, excessive exercise was recognized as a form of purging that some people with bulimia engage in. To qualify as excessive,

◆ What Happens to a Person With Bulimia?

Okay. You don't want a lecture about what can happen when you vomit or use laxatives or other medications. You just want the information so that you can make your own decision. No lecture, just the facts.

◆ Your face can look fatter due to swollen, puffy skin and enlarged salivary (parotid) glands.

◆ You can permanently destroy the enamel on your teeth and you may need expensive dental work.

◆ Your stomach can send acid into the esophagus, causing heartburn or ulcers.

◆ Your stomach or esophagus can burst from vomiting. You can die from this.

◆ After eating and purging for several days, your heart may race as if you are sprinting.

◆ You may feel dizzy when you stand up.

◆ You may feel like you wake up with a hangover every morning.

◆ You may steal food and are at heightened risk for drug and alcohol abuse.

◆ Your digestive system may never be the same and you may have years of feeling bloated and swollen in the stomach. You may have difficulty with your bowel movements.

◆ Your menstrual cycle will be out of balance and you can miss periods or have periods that last for weeks. This can affect your ability to have children.

◆ You are at risk for the female athlete triad, because if you miss periods for three months or more you may develop a stress fracture or long-term irreversible osteoporosis.

◆ Your life will be consumed by the habit of eating and then purging, so that you don't think of anything else.

exercise must be done compulsively, purely to burn extra calories and undo the effects of overeating or bingeing. The extra exercise is done not for fun or fitness or training, but solely with the goal of burning calories. For example, a woman who counts calories strictly and goes over her predetermined amount will run long enough to burn up the extra calories. The abuse of exercise to burn unwanted calories makes this another purging behavior. You may recognize people who over-exercise for this purpose. To qualify as having bulimia, these people will also have all of the other criteria, but they use exercise instead of a purging method like vomiting or laxative abuse. What is the problem with this? In a nutshell, excessive exercise leads to injuries, a compulsion to exercise to the exclusion of other activities, and the other psychological problems of bulimia, such as depression and low self-esteem.

To summarize, the sad fact about the purging methods used regularly by people with bulimia is that these are self-inflicted, abusive behaviors. Out of desperation to lose weight, women use these harmful, often painful, and embarrassing behaviors. These techniques do not result in effective weight loss because they only cause dehydration. Most people with the disorder would like to stop these behaviors and they hide them as much as is possible. But they find that stopping is very difficult; they have a compulsion to continue to use them to try to control or lose weight. These purging methods lead to serious medical and psychological problems.

OVERCOMING BULIMIA

Because bulimia is a multifaceted disorder, there are many reasons people get into this cycle. Thus, there are different approaches to treating it. Some researchers believe psychological problems come after dieting, a change that was demonstrated in the semistarvation studies mentioned in chapter 2. Others believe there are predisposing personalities and a psychological profile that precede the bulimia. Some researchers have linked bulimia (particularly the bingeing aspect) to a deficiency of brain chemical known as serotonin. Bulimia has been found to respond to drugs that increase the levels of serotonin in the brain. See chapter 7 for more specifics about treating bulimia.

Bulimia is also thought of as an addictive disorder in which the person is addicted to the binge-purge cycle. Like other forms of addiction, bulimia may be a person's way of manifesting self-treatment for some other form of pain or distress. Food, or the act of bingeing and purging, becomes a self-treatment—a sedative, or a stress reliever, like alcohol or drugs. However, unlike other addictive substances, food cannot be avoided. A person with bulimia cannot stop eating.

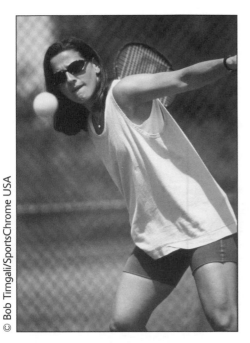

Exercise for fun, for fitness, or for training purposes—not as a means of burning calories.

Learning to eat normally is incredibly difficult to do. She may have the all-or-none thinking typical of alcoholics: if I cannot avoid food, I might as well eat a lot and then get rid of it by purging. A high rate of drug and alcohol use is also common in people with bulimia.

People who have bulimia usually attempt to hide most of their behavior. That is why we call this chapter "Out of the Kitchen and Into the Closet." Bulimia is their secret. Whether they consider it shameful or a source of secret pride, many people will hide this habit for years. One prominent athletic trainer who now counsels athletes with eating disorders told a national audience that she hid her bulimia for 15 years from her teammates, her husband, her children, and her coworkers. When she was fed up with the behavior, she finally came in for treatment. We also saw this in Jessica's story.

People with bulimia often shoplift food. They may be in financial difficulties because of the amount of money it takes to fund a binge-purge habit. One patient I cared for took 50 laxatives a day. The majority of her time and income went into trips to buy these laxatives at many different stores and to buy the food for her binges. She had to take out student loans and ran up large credit card bills.

It is surprising that there are almost no long-term outcome studies in the medical or psychological treatment of eating disorders in women, and none at all for female athletes. In my experience, women with long-standing bulimia find it very difficult to stop these practices without professional help. They may stop for awhile and think they have it under control. But they return to overeating and purging when there is a period of stress or pressure to lose weight. The women who have recovered have entered treatment that deals with not only the eating behavior but also the underlying psychological problems that lead women to use self-inflicted abusive behaviors. Psychological therapy works best when it is directed at building self-esteem, helping the woman develop a positive body image, and dealing with underlying depression or a history of being abused. We still have a great deal to learn about the best way to help athletic women with bulimia heal. The female athlete triad has just recently been recognized. We are presently in the early stages of understanding many of its components.

However, encouraging someone with bulimia to get help can make a tremendous difference in her life. Three of the women you met in this chapter, Jessica, Rosie, and Eileen, got caught in the cycle of bulimia. They suffered physical and emotional problems for many years. They were able to break this destructive cycle by seeking help and dealing with not only the bulimic behavior but also other underlying issues. Bulimia is a very treatable disorder, but recovering takes time, serious effort, and courage. If you or someone you care about suffers from bulimia, get the care you need.

Rosie began treatment for bulimia with me in the student health center. She told me that she had started dieting and vomiting when she was 12 and was in a gymnastics camp. She was targeted as one of the "fatties," and she was told to eat only salad and four ounces of skinless chicken a day. She and the other "fatties" were not allowed to leave their rooms at night, but they learned how to sneak out and get food. They were starving! One night after eating a whole box of Oreos, she and two friends forced themselves to throw up. She continued this practice during the entire camp, never telling her parents. When she went home after camp, she told me that her life seemed to revolve around hidden eating and vomiting and gymnastics practice. She thought about telling her mother once when she saw blood in the toilet after throwing up, but her parents were going through a divorce and she did not want to worry her mother. When she went to college, she continued vomiting and also started to use laxatives. She had episodes of dizziness, a racing heart, and often felt dizzy on the balance beam. She was in denial that any of these symptoms were caused by her bulimia. Then she was hospitalized for abdominal pain. She had tried to vomit a half-eaten bagel and it had gotten stuck in her esophagus. She had such severe pain that she nearly passed out.

The doctors had to look down her throat into the esophagus with a specialized tube. They found a lot of irritation and bleeding. They told her she had almost died because she could have torn her esophagus. When she was discharged from the hospital, she agreed to see me on a regular basis. She had been really frightened by this hospitalization. She actually found it a relief to be talking about the bulimia because it had been running her life for years. Her physical examination and blood tests showed that she was anemic and had low amounts of potassium from her daily vomiting habit. We worked on her eating small amounts of food during the day and replacing her potassium with a tablet. She also started iron pills and multiple vitamins.

She decided to tell her parents and to also see a team psychologist. She found it hard to change her daily habits of not eating and then vomiting after a small dinner, but she was able to eat small amounts during the day. She decided to take a semester off from gymnastics. With the support of the team psychologist, she told her teammates about what had really happened to her. Eight years of secrecy came tumbling down in a very emotional team meeting that the team psychologist led. Rosie's teammates were all very supportive of her, telling her how much they loved her and respected her. They also had their own struggles with weight, and some of them had bulimia. The team members decided to set up a peer program to help each other with the weight issues. Rosie continued in individual therapy and regained some of her health. She greatly decreased her vomiting and no longer felt dizzy. She resumed gymnastics at college and was able to perform better on the beam once she was no longer so dehydrated.

You can learn more about prevention and treatments for bulimia in chapters 7 and 8. But first, get to know the effects both anorexia and bulimia have on your menstrual cycles (chapter 5) and bone density (chapter 6).

WHAT JESSICA'S, EILEEN'S, AND ROSIE'S EXPERIENCES TEACH US

All three women developed bulimia in fairly common ways. Eileen's behavior was triggered by a binge, while Rosie and Jessica started on the road to bulimia using starvation diets. As is typical in women with eating disorders, they hid their behavior from close family, friends, coaches and teammates. Although upset by being trapped in the cycle of bingeing and purging, they were unable to stop their bulimic behavior on their own. All three women developed medical and psychological problems and only came to treatment after serious health scares. There are many warning signs of and risk factors for bulimia.

Bulimia often starts with dieting, which then leads to overeating.

Although not everyone who diets develops bulimia, Jessica and Rosie were pressured into starvation diets in mistaken attempts to improve their performance. Active women should not diet during training or competition.

Action to take: Educate yourself and your friends about unrealistic diets and their harmful effects. Get a professional opinion about your weight goals and advice from a nutritionist about how best to reach them. If, like Rosie, a coach or trainer puts you on a starvation diet or insists you lose weight, tell your parents and medical authorities at once.

Purging behaviors do not work to cause the loss of "real" weight. Rather, they induce dehydration and loss of water weight.

Jessica and Rosie became frustrated when their attempts to lose weight failed because the methods they used were ineffective. Their weight loss was temporary and returned immediately after they rehydrated. They experienced the symptoms of dehydration such as dizziness, racing heart rate, and reduced performance.

Action to take: It is essential to understand that the purging methods do not work. If you are unclear on this point, reread pages 96 to 102 in this chapter that explain how the purging methods remove water and essential electrolytes instead of calories. If you use these techniques, do not blame poor performance on your weight. Read pages 94 to 96 to understand how dehydration impairs performance.

Certain women are at more risk for developing bulimia.

People with depression, poor body image or self-esteem, a history of abuse, or pressures to "make weight" seem to be at most risk.

Action to take: Early recognition and treatment of risk factors (such as poor body image) coupled with avoidance of extreme dieting can help prevent bulimia. Education about the factors that influence active women to develop bulimia can help reduce the pressure they feel to live up to unrealistic weight standards.

Bulimia is often a "smoke alarm," a cry for help for the underlying problems. It is best treated by addressing the underlying issues.

Eileen often used bingeing and purging as a way of managing stress. If she had a difficult day at work, she felt better after eating her favorite food and throwing it up. When she finally saw a doctor for help with insomnia, the doctor guided her to therapy with a psychologist. After dealing with the things that were really bothering her and developing other stress reduction strategies, she had fewer urges to overeat.

Action to take: Learn to recognize when you are under stress or depressed. Be honest with your feelings and write them in a journal, or see a counselor instead of turning to food. If you know you have some serious underlying issues, such as a history of abuse or significant depression, seek care now.

Most people with bulimia are embarrassed by their behavior and want to stop, but because of the compulsive, addictive nature, they find it almost impossible to stop on their own.

Jessica and Rosie both thought they were in control when they were not. They did not realize the addictive potential of their behavior, and although Rosie wanted to stop using laxatives, she found she couldn't. Often, friends and family of someone with bulimia do not understand why she cannot just stop this dangerous behavior. They also do not understand the difficulty of changing this cycle.

Action to take: Realize that just wanting to stop, while a great start, is not enough. Think about another repetitive behavior that people might want to stop, even one as mundane as nail-biting. Almost everyone has found they can't just stop. They need to take certain steps that involve behavior modification and stress management. The same is true for bulimia. Most people need to seek professional care (see chapter 7) to deal with the substantial issues that drive their disorder.

Pressure from coaches and others to meet strict weight standards and weigh-ins often prompts athletes to experiment with bulimic practices. Vulnerable athletes, or those with recurrent weight pressures, may get trapped in the cycle of bulimia.

At age 12, Rosie was told by her gymnastics coach that she was a "fattie" and was put on a starvation diet at gymnastics camp. Jessica faced mandatory weigh-ins for the swim team and wearing skimpy uniforms.

Action to take: Coaches and other professionals should be educated about the impact mandatory weigh-ins, strict weight standards and body composition testing have on the health and psyches of young women. They also can benefit from courses about nutrition and effective weight management. If you are subjected to pressure from your coach to lose weight, check with medical personnel and a nutritionist to make sure your weight goal is reasonable and can be reached safely.

What Jessica, Rosie, and Eileen Did Right

♦ Sought help from professionals
♦ Realized and accepted that modifying a longstanding behavior takes considerable time and effort
♦ Learned to deal directly with emotional issues
♦ Learned to reject unrealistic weight expectations

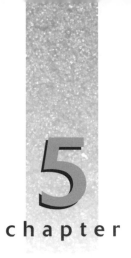

5
chapter

The Power
of Your Period:
Amenorrhea

Although most people have heard about eating disorders, many have not heard much about amenorrhea—the absence of menstrual periods. That may be because there is little discussion about menstrual cycles. Even when menstruation is talked about, the discussions are often filled with myths and misinformation.

Amenorrhea is another component of the female athlete triad (though it can also occur independently of the triad). Within the context of the triad, amenorrhea develops due to the energy drain caused by disordered eating. Women with amenorrhea are also at risk for osteoporosis, another consequence of the triad (see chapter 6). Some people erroneously believe that amenorrhea can be a normal or expected consequence of athletic training, something that active women should not worry about. Wrong. Stopping menstrual periods is not normal, but rather is a signal that something is going wrong in your body.

When **Deborah's** menstrual periods stopped, she thought she was finally getting into shape and was ready for her high school senior cross country season. Many of her friends also stopped having their periods when they started increasing the intensity of their cross country workouts. They welcomed the convenience of not having to worry about getting their periods. They had never heard there was anything wrong with not menstruating; it was just part of being an athlete in training.

Rowena, a former college gymnast, was 27 years old and had been married for two years. After competing in college gymnastics, she worked as an aerobics instructor. She and her husband were trying to have a baby, but she did not have regular menstrual cycles. She had never really had normal periods. She didn't start her periods until she was 17, and then she usually had two or three periods a year at the most. Without a normal cycle, her doctors told her that it would be very difficult for her to get pregnant and that she might have to use fertility drugs.

You may recognize the experiences of Rowena and Deborah and wonder what is so bad about amenorrhea. After all, it's a relief not to have monthly menstrual flow, cramps, and premenstrual syndrome (PMS). But amenorrhea means that your ovaries are not functioning as they should. As a result, you do not release an egg each month and you lack adequate levels of the ovarian hormones estrogen, progesterone, and testosterone. These hormones enable you to build bone, grow hair, have glowing skin, and enjoy sex. They provide vaginal lubrication during sexual arousal and improve your libido, or your interest in sex.

There are several changes that can occur in the menstrual cycle whether you are physically active or not. These include the following:

- ◆ Primary amenorrhea or delayed menarche—not starting your periods by age 16
- ◆ Oligomenorrhea—irregular menstrual periods, in which bleeding occurs at erratic intervals of 12 to 90 days
- ◆ Secondary amenorrhea—complete absence of menstrual periods for three months or more

Each of these conditions can be caused by a wide variety of medical problems. Some menstrual cycle changes are associated with exercise; some are not. However, we do know that exercise by itself does not cause changes in the menstrual cycle, nor is amenorrhea a normal consequence of exercise. Rather amenorrhea is a red flag, a warning that something is seriously wrong with the body. Moreover, research has convincingly connected the effects of amenorrhea to serious stress fractures and osteoporosis. Sports medicine experts now see amenorrhea as a telling sign of overtraining or energy imbalance. Impaired nutrition, energy drain, eating disorders, hormonal imbalances, and stress are the most common underlying causes. Amenorrhea is often the first diagnosed symptom of the female athlete triad.

Read further to find out more about amenorrhea's effects on your fitness, your performance, and your long-term health, sexuality, and fertility. If you or a friend or teammate has amenorrhea, you will learn what to do about it. First, let's briefly review the phases of a normal menstrual cycle.

YOUR HEALTHY MENSTRUAL CYCLE

Often there are more questions than answers about the changes in an active woman's menstrual cycle. Current research on active women and their menstrual cycles parallels what we have learned from talking to women. Each woman has her own experience of her menstrual cycles. For some it is a breeze, with just the temporary inconvenience of using tampons or pads. For others it is a time of uncomfortable physical feelings like bloating, nausea, diarrhea, and painful cramps. One woman may train as hard as her teammates, but she stops menstruating whereas they don't. What is true for one woman may not be true for her friend or her sister. Though there are variations among women, when something changes in your menstrual cycle it is a sign that you should visit your doctor for a medical evaluation.

Monthly menstrual bleeding is the most obvious sign of the workings of a woman's complex reproductive system. Actually, the menstrual bleeding is just one part of a process regulated by the master gland of the body, the hypothalamus. The hypothalamus is like the thermostat of the body. Recall its role in regulating body weight and the set point discussed in chapter 1. It also plays a role in starting the changes of puberty. The job of the hypothalamus is not only to send signals to direct the menstrual cycle but also to keep the body's energy in balance. The hypothalamus will not send the signals unless everything is just right. Its job is to make sure the body has enough energy to sustain the reproductive cycle and a possible pregnancy. You may not be at all interested in getting pregnant, but the hypothalamus doesn't know that. It has been programmed to be ready to reproduce the species. If it senses that the body is energy deficient, it will take action to conserve energy and protect the body from harm. How does it do this? The hypothalamus receives and integrates information from inside and outside of the body. It ensures that everything is as it should be before sending the signals that direct the reproductive system to complete the menstrual cycle.

In the normal menstrual cycle, when the hypothalamus recognizes that everything is in balance, it sends a signal hormone called GnRH (gonadotrophin releasing hormone) to the other master gland of the body, the pituitary. The pituitary then sends signals to the ovary. The pituitary's signals are called FSH (follicle stimulating hormone) and LH (luteinizing hormone). The ovary's job is to respond to these signals by making two hormones, estrogen and progesterone, and releasing an egg.

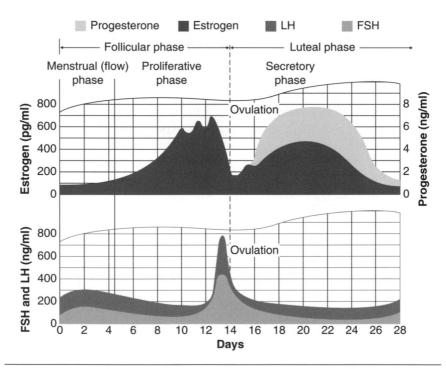

Figure 5.1 The phases of the menstrual cycle as illustrated by the changes in progesterone and estrogen (top) and FSH and LH (bottom). Menstrual bleeding marks the start of the follicular phase while ovulation marks the beginning of the luteal phase.

Reprinted, by permission, from J.H. Wilmore and D.L. Costill, 1999, *Physiology of Sports and Exercise*, 2nd ed. (Champaign, IL: Human Kinetics), 588.

The menstrual cycle has four phases (figure 5.1): the follicular phase, ovulation, the luteal phase, and menstrual bleeding. In the follicular phase, FSH from the pituitary causes the ovary to develop eggs and make the hormone estrogen. Estrogen acts on the uterus to start a lining. As the eggs in the ovary develop and levels of estrogen rise, the pituitary gland senses these changes. It then sends a second hormonal signal (LH) to the ovary to release the egg—ovulation.

A woman may have symptoms during ovulation. She may notice that she has a pain on one of her lower sides that lasts for a few days. Her body temperature will go up a few tenths of a degree.

The luteal phase occurs after ovulation and lasts until menstrual bleeding begins. This phase of the cycle consistently averages 14 days. The luteal phase prepares a woman's body for pregnancy. At the beginning of this phase, the egg is released, and it travels from the ovary through the Fallopian tubes toward the uterus. The ovary then produces a second hormone, progesterone. Progesterone, along with estrogen, develops the uterine lining further so that it is ready to receive a fertilized egg. If the egg is not fertilized, then the ovary stops making estrogen and progesterone 14 days after ovulation. The decline in levels of estrogen and progesterone causes the uterine lining to break down, and the result is menstrual bleeding. During the luteal phase, a woman may experience breast tenderness, bloating, increase in acne, mood swings, and mild weight gain because of the production of progesterone. These symptoms are called molimina, and they are indicative of a normal menstrual cycle. They usually disappear as soon as the menstrual flow begins.

There are some athletic women who do not produce an egg or adequate levels of progesterone during the luteal phase. They still have a fairly regular menstrual flow, but they do not have the premenstrual symptoms. This is a condition called luteal phase deficiency. The woman generally does not recognize this as abnormal because she has a regular menstrual flow. However, there are some reports that luteal phase deficiency can lead to inadequate bone formation or to difficulty becoming pregnant. If you think you might have this condition, you need to have your hormone levels checked by a physician for accurate diagnosis and treatment.

The length of time between periods in a normal menstrual cycle can be 23 to 38 days, though this pattern may vary and still be considered normal. The usual duration of flow is four to six days, but bleeding that lasts two to eight days can be normal and does not indicate a problem. The amount of flow can vary from month to month and can be as little as 40 cc (10 teaspoons) or as much as 400 cc (100 teaspoons). Women who bleed heavily lose more than just menstrual blood; they also lose more iron, a mineral contained in the blood. These women are at a higher risk for iron-poor blood—otherwise known as anemia. It is because of menstrual blood loss that women need almost twice as much iron as men, 15 to 18 mg a day. See table 5.1 for the amounts of iron that regular serving sizes of various foods.

If women do not get enough iron in their diets, they do not have the iron to make new red blood cells. Red blood cells are needed to carry oxygen from the lungs to the exercising tissues. If the red-blood-

Table 5.1
Iron Content of Commonly Eaten Foods

Food	Quantity	Iron (mg) [18mg = 100% RDA]
Animal sources*		
Liver, chicken	4 ounces cooked	9
Lean steak	4 ounces	3
Turkey (dark meat)	4 ounces	2
Lamb	4 ounces	3
Pork	4 ounces	1
Oysters, raw	6 medium	6
Shrimp	12 large	2
Chicken breast	4 ounces	1
Fish (haddock or salmon)	4 ounces	1
Tuna (light)	3 ounces	1
Egg	1 large	1
Fruits and juices		
Prune juice	8 ounces	3
Dried apricots	5 halves	0.8
Dried dates	10	1
Raisins	1/3 cup	1
Vegetables and legumes**		
Kidney beans	1 cup	6

Refried beans	1 cup	4.5
Spinach	1/2 cup cooked	3
Tofu	1/4 cake	2
Peas	1/2 cup	1
Broccoli	1/2 cup	1
Dairy products		
Skim milk	1 cup	0.1
Cheddar cheese	1 ounce	0.2
Grains		
Cereal, Total	1 cup	18
Raisin Bran, Kellogg's	3/4 cup	18
Cream of Wheat	1 cup	9
Pasta, enriched	1 cup cooked	2
Bread, enriched	1 slice	1
Brown rice	1 cup cooked	1
Other sources		
Brewer's yeast	1 ounce	5
Black strap molasses	1 tablespoon	3.5
Wheat germ	1/4 cup	2

*Animal sources of iron are absorbed best (except for iron from eggs).

**Vegetable sources of iron are poorly absorbed.

Nutrient data from J. Pennington, 1992, *Bowes and Church's Food Values of Portions Commonly Used*, 16th ed. (Philadelphia: Lippincott.) Reprinted, by permission, from N. Clark, 1997.

cell count is lower, the oxygen-carrying capacity of the blood is lower, and athletic performance will decrease, resulting in sluggishness in practice or competition.

PRIMARY AMENORRHEA

You remember puberty, don't you? That awkward time when your body changed in ways you couldn't predict or control and that you probably did not want to happen. Strange things occurred, like

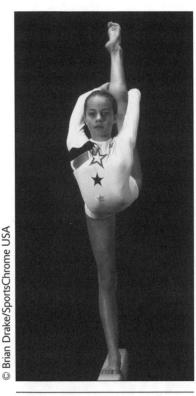

© Brian Drake/SportsChrome USA

Athletes who participate in sports such as gymnastics often experience puberty later than other girls.

sudden growth spurts, acne, breast buds, and weight gain. And after all this, along came menarche—your first menstrual period.

Both boys and girls go through dramatic body changes as they grow into adulthood. The changes in boys are caused by the principal male hormone, testosterone. Testosterone directs the development of male pattern body hair on the face and causes boys to develop more acne, to become taller, and to have more muscle mass and stronger bones than girls. Testosterone is known as an anabolic hormone, meaning that it acts to build and strengthen muscle and bone. Because women have very low levels of testosterone, they do not develop as much muscle or bone tissue as men. Estrogen is the dominant female hormone. Estrogen directs the body to develop breasts and to distribute body fat around the hips and thighs. It is an essential hormone that also helps build bone, nourishes skin and vaginal tissue, lowers cholesterol, and fuels sexual drive.

These hormonally induced body changes also affect physical performance. Before puberty, boys and girls are pretty much equal in terms of athletic performance. After puberty, however, a boy gains more muscle mass and strength, has stronger bones, and has a larger heart and lungs and less body fat compared to a girl of the same height. After puberty, a girl has a higher percentage of body fat and relatively less muscle and bone mass.

Researchers first thought that a girl had to be a certain weight or body fat percentage to start having her periods. However, further study has shown that weight or body fat alone are not the sole factors that determine puberty or menarche. Rather, the chief influence on the timing of puberty is genetic. That means that if your parents experienced a later puberty, you are likely to be a late bloomer as well. Other factors, including stress, nutrition, and exercise, can also influence the timing of puberty. Because the master gland of the body, the hypothalamus, controls the events of puberty, anything that disrupts the function of the hypothalamus—restrictive diets, poor nutrition, eating disorders, and stress—can delay it. Medical problems such as diabetes, brain tumors, thyroid disorders, and other hormone problems can also delay puberty.

Diane is a 4'10" gymnast who is 14 years and three months old. She has not yet started her period, but she isn't worried, because no one else on her team has started either. In fact, she dreads going through puberty, because she thinks it will be the end of her gymnastics career. All her teammates talk about wanting to stay small so that they can still be good in gymnastics. Diane has a rigorous training schedule, training five to seven days a week, three to four hours a day, year round at a local club. She lives for competition and wants to go to the Olympics. She is concerned about her weight and only eats low-fat foods.

Diane's parents were worried that she hadn't started having her periods yet. They remembered her older sister starting her period when she was 12 years old. When they took Diane to the family doctor, she checked Diane's growth chart and found that her growth had slowed. Diane had grown only a half-inch and had gained two pounds in the past year. She had started seeing some breast development by age 12½, but she did not get any body hair. Diane seemed to have stopped growing and developing in the middle of puberty. Diane thought she was fine and was not worried about any problem. The doctor ran some blood tests to check for hormonal or medical problems and suggested she see a nutritionist. Diane was angry at her parents for making her go to the doctor and resolved to work out harder and eat less so that she would never start her period.

Diane's reaction to growing up is not unusual. Many girls who are committed to a sport like gymnastics, which values small, lean, compact physiques, do not want their bodies to change or to start having periods. However, it is a fact of life that we go through puberty. As previously noted, the orderly parade of events of puberty is controlled by many factors, including heredity, nutrition, medical health, family size, stressors, and physical activity. Therefore, if a girl experiences delayed puberty, all factors must be evaluated. The place to start the evaluation is with a pediatrician or physician. Usually girls have been tracked for the growth and developmental stages of puberty by their doctors, who keep height and weight records on standardized growth charts to see if girls are developing normally.

Delayed Puberty in Active Girls

Girls who naturally experience a later puberty are more likely to have the body type preferred in activities such as gymnastics and ballet. Although there is currently not enough evidence to support that childhood participation in a sport delays puberty in girls, researchers are looking into the possibility. Only recently have large numbers of young girls begun strenuous training before puberty, so answering this question will take one or two decades of careful tracking of girls and their pubertal development. There is evidence, however, that inadequate nutrition or eating disorders can impair growth and delay puberty. Because many factors determine the timing of puberty, each girl must be individually assessed by a physician experienced in this area.

Questions and Answers About Puberty

Q. Has my development or puberty begun early, late, or on time?

A. If you start to develop breast tissue by age 8, you may have started puberty too early and should be seen by a physician for an evaluation of precocious puberty. If you have not had any breast development by age 12 or 13 at the latest, you should be checked for delayed puberty.

Q. Can I predict when my menstrual cycles will start?

A. An estimate is that your first menstrual cycle (known as menarche) will come 30 to 36 months after your breasts begin to develop. The average age of menarche is 12 to 12.9 years. Normal girls can have their menarche as young as 10 years, 8 months of age or as late as age 14.

Q. When should I worry if my menstrual periods do not start?

A. If you started breast development but did not start having periods by age 16, you should be seen by a doctor for a medical checkup. If you are 14 and have not yet begun breast development and have not had a menstrual period, you should also see a physician.

Q. Is there any way to tell how tall I will be?

A. Height is genetically determined. Maximum height is generally reached about one to two years after your first menstrual period. You can expect to grow one to six inches (an average of three inches) taller after the date of your menarche.

After **Diane** went for a medical evaluation, she told her team-mates and coach what the doctor and nutritionist had said: she needed more calcium in her diet, and they were concerned that she had not started to menstruate. She shared a handout on calcium, and the whole team agreed to have high-calcium snacks during breaks. The coach brought in yogurt, nonfat milk, and calcium-fortified orange juice. A few of her teammates did the three-day diet recall the nutritionist wanted Diane to do along with her.

Diane also had her bone age measured by having her left wrist and hand X-rayed. This test compared the age of her skeleton to her real age. The results of all the tests showed that Diane was not getting enough calories and that her growth had stopped. Diane and her family were willing to make changes to improve Diane's nutrition. Although she did not really like the thought of getting her period, she did want someday to have children.

Diane gained four pounds over the next three months with a healthy diet and added snacks. She found her energy was better. She was doing more moves in her tumbling routine than she had ever done. Six months later she had grown another inch and gained another four pounds. She looked lean and fit. A year later, when she was 16, she finally started her periods and had breasts and hips. She still enjoyed gymnastics. She remembered the time when she had not wanted to get her period and grow up. She had wanted to be carefree and fly around the gymnastics bars like a bird. Now that she was heavier, she didn't fly around the bars as fast, but she felt strong and in control and looked forward to her last year of high school, to dating, and to college.

Puberty is a difficult time for girls. Some girls start the battle of control over their bodies at this transition time. The battle takes the form of restricting "enemy" foods and trying to control everything they eat to offset weight gain and changes in their bodies. Some girls develop anorexia (chapter 3), bulimia (chapter 4), delayed menarche or amenorrhea, and become candidates for osteoporosis (chapter 6). They lose control of their health by attempting to control their bodies. These women become too thin to win, too weak to compete, and eventually they can suffer stress fractures that force them to take time off from training to heal. With the support of family, friends, coaches, and doctors, girls can make the transition to puberty successfully. With the new-found strength of an adult body, they go on to become winners and champions.

Risks of Primary Amenorrhea

Why should anyone care whether she goes through puberty "on time" or not? After all, many girls do not want to go through puberty at all! The first reason is that a delay in menarche may be the only sign you see of a serious underlying medical problem. It can be a marker of a hormone imbalance, a brain tumor, inadequate nutrition, or an early eating disorder. The earlier these conditions are recognized, the better the outcome. If normal maturation is delayed there is cause for great concern, because we are all programmed, like it or not, to mature into adults.

In addition to the concern about an underlying medical condition, there is the possibility that primary amenorrhea may also cause early weakening of the bones, or osteoporosis, another component of the female athlete triad. If a girl does not start having her period, she is not getting the normal amount of estrogen that is necessary to build her skeleton. The few studies that evaluated the risks of primary amenorrhea in athletic girls confirm this concern for bone health. One longitudinal study on professional ballerinas with delayed menarche found that they had a significant increased risk for scoliosis (curvature of the spine), stress fractures, and complete bone fractures (figure 5.2).

What is happening to these women? If the body does not begin menstruation, the skeleton is not exposed to normal amounts of the female hormones necessary for it to develop. Remember, your skeleton is doing a great deal of growing during the years of puberty. If something goes wrong during this phase, it may not be correctable. (See chapter 6 for more information about the growth of the normal skeleton during puberty). If you start menstruation four years later than you normally would have because of inadequate nutrition, does your skeleton lose four years of bone mass, or does it catch up? The answer to that question is not known. More research is needed to see how significant primary amenorrhea is to bone development. While we wait for more research, it is important that all girls with primary amenorrhea be evaluated and treated and any health risks reduced.

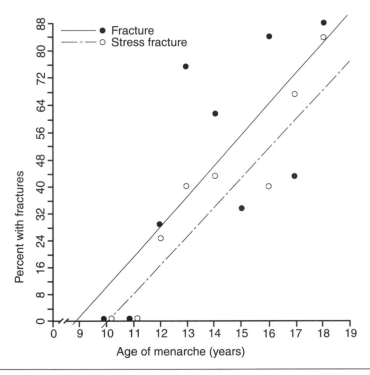

Figure 5.2 Relation between age of menarche and the percentage of subects with fractures or stress fractures.

Reprinted, with permission, from M.P. Warren, J. Brooks-Gunn, L.H. Hamilton, L. Fiske Warren, and W.G. Hamilton, 1986, "Scoliosis and fractures in young ballet dancers: Relation to delayed menarche and secondary amenorrhea," *New England Journal of Medicine* 314:1348-1353.

SECONDARY AMENORRHEA AND OLIGOMENORRHEA

Secondary amenorrhea occurs when a woman who has reached menarche stops having menstrual periods for three months or more. Oligomenorrhea refers to few or irregular menstrual periods. Oligomenorrhea may be a precursor to amenorrhea. Like amenorrhea, it is a marker that something is wrong. The periods may be at irregular intervals, varying between 21 and 90 days, with usually fewer than six periods per year.

Why would an athletic woman's periods change? Possibly because of an underlying medical problem or an energy drain. Any woman who experiences a change in her menstrual cycle should be checked for underlying medical problems. If none are found, then the change may be due to the hypothalamus sensing an energy drain. The hypothalamus, the thermostat of the body, assesses the body's overall energy status and senses that there is too much energy going out and not enough coming in. It deals with this problem by temporarily "turning off" the reproductive system (lowering levels of the pituitary hormones and ovarian hormones) as a strategy to conserve energy. The three main types of hypothalamic amenorrhea are

- stress-related—diagnosed by life changes, high stress level;
- exercise-associated—due to a history of increased amounts of physical training; and
- eating disordered—due to inadequate nutrition.

A fourth subtype of hypothalamic amenorrhea, caused by a growth or tumor in the brain that destroys the hypothalamus, is very rare and is not related to the triad.

Amenorrhea can be caused by a variety of medical problems. So, how can a woman tell what caused her amenorrhea? Is it due to a hormonal imbalance, a brain tumor, exercise, disordered eating, or even pregnancy? Finding the cause requires a thorough evaluation by a physician or other clinically trained expert. Only by taking a careful history, doing a physical examination, and checking the results of blood tests can a clinician accurately determine the cause of amenorrhea.

If no other medical condition is found, the amenorrhea is likely due to the hypothalamus temporarily turning off the reproductive system because of a perceived energy drain. How and why does the hypothalamus sense energy drain or stress? This protective system has been in place in our bodies for millions of years to protect women from getting pregnant during starvation or energy deficiency. When the energy drain was gone, a prehistoric woman's menstrual cycles and ability to have children returned. Today's athletic woman lives in a very different world from our Stone Age ancestors', but our reproductive systems are still programmed to stop or slow down if there is an energy imbalance. For modern women, the energy drain is often caused by inadequate nutrition, the energy expenditure of exercise or stress, or a combination of all three.

Stress results from anything that demands energy. It can be something good or bad. A heavy workload in athletics or in your job results in stress because of the mental and physical energy your body demands to fuel these activities. Travel, work, competition, and erratic sleep add to stress by also depleting your energy. If the increased stress is accompanied by inadequate rest and nutrition, the energy drain is further magnified. The body responds to stress by producing a variety of hormones, including one called cortisol. High levels of cortisol affect the master gland, the hypothalamus, and signal it to store fat and conserve energy. Recently, it was discovered that fat cells send a hormone signal called leptin to the hypothalamus. It is felt that leptin indicates the body's energy intake level. Preliminary work suggests that leptin may be one signal that tells the body it has adequate energy stores and is ready to begin puberty. Leptin may also be a factor in secondary amenorrhea. These complex systems are in place to inform the body of its energy status. The hypothalamus, that wise thermostat, is informed of the amount of available energy in the body and can recognize an energy drain from stress or poor nutrition. It conserves energy by stopping menstruation while the energy drain and stress are still present. Studies on both sedentary women and athletic women have found that just a few days of intense stress, particularly if associated with inadequate food intake, can suppress the hypothalamus.

At the student health clinic where I work, it is very common for both first-year students and graduate students going through PhD exams to stop having their periods for a while. For these students, stress is the energy drain of moving 3,000 miles away from home, living in a dorm room with two strangers as roommates, and late-night studying. For other women, working full-time, having a child, trying to lose weight after delivery, and relationship stresses can all contribute to an energy deficit. Although stress or energy drain is the most likely cause of one type of amenorrhea, there are other medical conditions that can cause a woman's period to stop. Every woman who stops menstruating or who experiences irregularities in her menstrual cycle should be seen by a physician.

In addition to life stresses, it has been recognized for over 50 years that when women train hard physically, some of them will stop having their periods. Women who competed in the Olympics in the 1950s and 60s commonly reported that their periods stopped when they were training and competing and resumed normally during the off-season. These athletes had normal pregnancies at the same rate as nonathletic women who did not stop having their periods. The type of amenorrhea associated with physical training has been called exercise-associated amenorrhea.

Deborah trained hard in the summer before her senior year of cross country, trying to qualify to make the state championship. She had missed a few menstrual periods during her junior year in high school, but during the fall of her senior year, she stopped having periods for three months. She was delighted, because one of those periods would have occurred during an important cross country meet. Most of the girls on her team also missed periods, and their coach told them it was no big deal and just a normal part of training hard.

For a long time, amenorrhea appeared to athletes, coaches, and trainers to be a normal and innocent change in athletes. Many women were delighted that their periods stopped. As my colleague Dr. Barney (Charlotte) Sanborn says, these women were shouting, "Amen for Amenorrhea!" In some circles it was even thought to be a mark of adequate training. You were considered "fit when it quit."

Then, in the early 1980s, researchers found that women runners with stress fractures were very likely to also have amenorrhea. Further work connected the stress fractures to amenorrhea and to the loss of bone mass. If enough bone loss occurs, the bones can become very susceptible to fracture—a condition called osteoporosis (see chapter 6). This finding perplexed researchers. Athletic women were supposed to have the strongest bones; after all, exercise—particularly weight-bearing exercise—acts to build bones, right? However, research showed that if a woman's menstrual periods stopped, she no longer had the female hormones needed to build strong bones. Exercise alone does not build bones without the presence of the female hormones, principally estrogen.

How common is it to stop having your period for three months or more? Surprisingly, it is fairly common. Among your nonathletic friends, 2 to 5 percent will stop having their periods during their teens or twenties. Most of the time this is due to a stressful situation and resolves when the stress is gone. Your athletic friends are more likely than your nonathletic friends to have episodes of amenorrhea. From 4 to 44 percent of physically active women report that they have stopped having their periods for three months or more. And if your friends are ballerinas, don't be surprised if most of them have stopped having periods. Questionnaire studies found that as many as 60 percent of professional ballerinas have stopped menstruating. Amenorrhea associated with exercise has been found in women training in all sports and activities, from aerobics and badminton to softball and tennis. However, though it is common, it is not normal, even if you are in peak fitness.

Amenorrhea and Performance

In our experience, most active women care a great deal about their performance, sometimes more than they care about their appearance. If you are a woman with exercise-associated amenorrhea, it is a warning sign that you are at risk for problems with your health and with your current and future athletic performance. Exercise-associated amenorrhea may be the first sign that you are doing too much training and are not giving your body the fuel it needs to balance this energy output. It puts you at risk for serious injuries such as stress fractures and results in poor concentration in the classroom, at work, and on the playing field. You must be willing to evaluate your training and your energy intake and to make the changes necessary to ensure that you are healthy and fit.

Recognizing Overtraining and Energy Drain

Think for a minute about how energetic you feel. Are you ready to go out and have a great workout or a fun night out on the town? Are you full of energy and enthusiasm when you wake up in the morning? How is your concentration and your ability to study or work hard? Are you eating and sleeping well, and are you interested and enthusiastic about your life? If you are not, you may have the early signs of overtraining. Overtraining is a state in which the body has done too much work and has not balanced that activity or workload with adequate sleep, rest, or nutrition to recover from it. The signs of overtraining include the following:

- Poor-quality sleep, restless sleep
- Feeling of staleness, lack of interest in physical training or daily activities
- Muscle soreness that does not recover after a night's rest
- Injuries that do not heal
- Elevated resting pulse (taken before getting out of bed)
- Fatigue
- Weight loss
- Decreased performance in school, at work, or in physical activity
- Frequent infections
- Mood disturbance: lack of interest, depression
- Amenorrhea

If you recognize four or more of these symptoms, you may be over-trained. The treatment for overtraining is to correct the energy drain and to allow some recovery time. Keeping a daily record of sleep patterns, physical activity, mood, heart rate before arising in the morning, nutritional intake, relaxation time, and injuries can help you get a handle on your energy balance and ensure that you are training optimally. Table 5.2 illustrates a completed training diary for Deborah. Chapter 7 includes a sample training diary that you can copy and use to monitor your own training (see table 7.1, page 228).

Measuring Your Energy Needs

You can calculate how much energy (calories) you use in a day. This will help you determine whether you are in deficit or not. The most

Table 5.2

Sample Training Diary for Deborah

Day	Monday	Tuesday	Wednesday
Resting pulse (before arising)	45	46	56
Sleep hours	5	6	3
Training pulse (maximum during training)	160	forgot	170
Fluid intake	2 bottles H$_2$0 2 cans sport drink	Same	2 bottles H$_2$0 1 juice 1 sport drink
Diet and caloric intake	bagel, apple, yogurt, salad, popcorn ? calories	bagel, banana, yogurt,pizza for study	cereal, sandwich, yogurt, juice
Mood	good	OK	tired
Any injuries	no	sore right hamstring	hamstring sore
Aerobic training	6 miles	2 mile warmup & down; 2 mile track intervals	2 miles easy 4 miles hard 2 miles easy
Strength training	none	none	15 pushups 100 ab curls
Other	—	had to study for midterm	—

accurate methods of measuring daily energy expenditure are used by professionals in a laboratory setting. However, scientists have developed equations you can use to estimate your daily energy expenditure. One of the easiest to use is shown on page 130. Remember that this is only an estimate.

Your daily energy expenditure is composed of two components:

1. Resting metabolic rate
2. Physical activity factors

Your resting metabolic rate (RMR) is the energy required to maintain your normal body functions, such as your body temperature, muscle activity, and heart rate. It is about two-thirds of your total

Thursday	Friday	Saturday	Sunday
52	50	50	52
6	4	6	10
180	—	150	140
?	3 bottles H$_2$O 1 sport drink	1 Diet cola 1 beer 2 bottles H$_2$O	3 bottles H$_2$O 2 cans sport drink
can't remember	bagel, sandwich, milk, rice bowl calories - 1200	cereal, apple, sandwich, cola, noodle soup, rice cakes	omelette, toast, o.j. calories - 1400
tired	OK	tired	tired
hamstring still sore	same soreness in hamstring	tight and sore hamstring	stopped to stretch right hamstring
2 miles track intervals & 2 miles easy	6 miles easy 2 miles tempo run	8 miles recovery on golf course	6 miles a.m. 8 miles p.m.
none	100 ab curls	15 pushups 100 ab curls	none
had to ice hamstring	iced hamstring	iced hamstring & took Advil	stretched

daily energy expenditure. You might remember from chapter 2 that muscle burns more calories at rest than fat does. Thus, the more muscle you have, the higher your resting metabolic rate is. Women have 5 to 10 percent less muscle than men, so they generally have a lower RMR. Physically trained women usually have more muscle—and thus a higher RMR—than untrained women. Women who are dieting have lower RMRs, and recent evidence suggests they may also have lower energy expenditures when they exercise. The equation to determine RMR was developed using total body weight (Sizer and Whitney; 2000).

Women: Resting Metabolic Rate in calories = 21.6 × (your weight in kilograms)
[Divide your weight in pounds by 2.2] [1 kilogram = 2.2 pounds]

In addition to the RMR, the other part of the equation is the physical activity factor (PAF). This measurement takes into account how active you are. A couch potato is not living at energy expenditure much higher than the resting metabolic rate. However, if you are a college sophomore who is on the swim team, taking 16 units of classes, working 10 hours a week as a waitress, and studying for midterms, your PAF factor is high! If you have two children, a job, a husband who expects you to do all the housework and cook all the meals, and you work out at the gym three times a week, your PAF factor is high! All of these things take energy, which equals stress (defined here as anything that requires energy).

To calculate your daily energy expenditure, use the equation given above to calculate your RMR. Then multiply that value by the appropriate PAF in table 5.3 (p. 131).

For example, in this chapter, Deborah is a 5'9", 124-pound (56.4 kg) high school cross country runner. She is very active, so she calculated her PAF as heavy (2.0). Her RMR is 21.6 × 56.4 kg (her weight in kilograms), which equals 1,218 calories a day. Her RMR (1218) times PAF (2) = 2,436 calories a day. If she did not meet this minimum daily energy need, by the end of a week, or a month, she would really be behind in her energy balance.

In Deborah's case, she is eating about 1,400 calories a day but needs about 2,400 calories. It is clear that she has an energy drain, and her symptoms of fatigue, amenorrhea, and an injury that does not heal are clearly related to this energy drain state.

Does the number of calories that Deborah needs surprise you? Does it seem high? It did to Deborah when these numbers were presented to her. She was shocked. To meet her daily energy needs and feel better, she clearly needs to make some changes. She needs to either add another 1,000 calories or decrease her energy expenditure. Sometimes the best way to get better is to do both; increase the daily calories and slightly reduce your training. Over a week or more there will be a measurable energy surplus.

Another consideration is what your energy equation has been for the past few weeks or months. If you have been consistently training seven days a week, skipping meals and running on empty, it will take more than just meeting your energy needs for a few days to correct your energy deficit. In addition to simply increasing calories, it is necessary to also get enough rest for your body to rebuild. Deborah had been in an energy deficit for at least six months, starting when she increased her running mileage and cut down on her food.

Correcting Energy Imbalance

Your energy comes mainly from food, plus whatever stored energy you have and the rest and relaxation you get. Stored energy is in the form of glycogen in the muscles, and fat. If you are very lean or are a chronic dieter, you may not have much of an energy reserve to meet your needs during times of stress, increased exercise, or high energy demand. If you are constantly on the go and have a lot of things to do, you may also have an energy deficit. It is important to get emotional support, relaxation, restful sleep, and take at least one day off a week from training to stay in energy balance. If you have good, supportive friends and family, and if you do something daily to renew and recharge your batteries, you are less likely to experience energy imbalance or to overtrain.

Table 5.3

Physical Activity Factors for Active Women

Activity level	Example	PAF
Sedentary	If you sit all day	1.3
Light	Such as a student or teacher	1.5
Moderate	If you exercise 1 hour, four to five times per week	1.6
Heavy	If you are an athlete in training	2.0
Exceptional	If you train intensely for many hours per day	2.2

Developed by Sheri Albert, MPH, RD, nutritionist at UCLA Arthur Ashe Student Health and Wellness Center. Adapted from formula and measures in Sizer and Whitney; 2000.

Many athletes have never been told the value and importance of taking days off during training. They mistakenly believe they must train seven days a week to reach their maximum potential. This is one way to never reach your maximum potential. In truth, a rest day allows you to recover and build the strength that you have worked so hard to achieve. Resting is as important to reaching your potential as all the exercise you perform to reach it. Rest allows your body to rebuild the muscles and consolidate the physiological gains from training. If you do not rest, you will most assuredly hit the wall of overtraining, simply because your body has not been given a chance to recover and rebuild again.

It is obvious that if you are in a state of constant energy drain, sooner or later something will give. This is when you feel tired, fall asleep in class, start losing weight, have injuries that do not heal, and develop amenorrhea. Recovering from this overtrained condition takes time. Take time off, relax, renew energy stores, and heal any injuries. How do you know when you have recovered? The symptoms of overtraining, such as a high resting pulse, amenorrhea, fatigue, and nonrestful sleep, are gone. You feel better, have a lower resting pulse, awaken in the morning refreshed, and your menstrual cycles come back. To see if you have recovered, use the daily training log and review the signs of overtraining again (see page 127). Make sure that your daily energy equation is in balance. Be patient, seek the advice of professionals if needed, and keep checking in with yourself.

Disordered Eating and Energy Drain

If you follow the idea of energy balance and do your own energy equation, you can see how important good nutrition is in avoiding energy imbalance. Think of an active woman who is dieting all the time or has developed disordered eating. Her energy availability from food is erratic or inadequate. If she has anorexia, she is constantly restricting her diet and is obviously lacking adequate energy intake. If she tries to use bulimic behavior to control her weight, one day she overeats, the next she starves. Another day, she might use laxatives and stay up all night with diarrhea, and then feel washed out the next day. Her body doesn't know if it is feasting or fasting.

Even without an eating disorder, some athletes get into energy imbalance accidentally. They are not consciously undereating nor do they have an eating disorder or body image distortion. Instead, some athletic women who do endurance training such as long-distance running, cycling, or swimming do not consume enough calories or take enough rest days to meet their high energy expenditures. A woman who runs up to 10 miles a day may be burning more than 4,000 calories and may not always keep up with these high caloric needs.

Now that you understand the concept of energy drain, you can make a list of factors that might put yourself, a teammate, or a friend at risk for energy imbalance, overtraining, poor performance, and amenorrhea. There is not one thing, or one amount of training or weight loss that will result in amenorrhea. Rather, it is a combination of factors that varies from person to person and from situation to situation. It is not weight loss alone or being below a certain body fat percentage. For example, on a cross country team, about half of the women might have amenorrhea. It is not always the thinnest athletes who will develop amenorrhea. Women who have had a past history of menstrual cycle changes or who have lost 10 pounds or more in the past year are more likely to have amenorrhea. Everyone has her own individual threshold for energy balance. If that balance is upset, then the body will take action to try to conserve energy or restore energy. The following list presents factors that increase one's risk for developing amenorrhea.

Risk Factors for Amenorrhea in Active Women

- ✦ Never been pregnant
- ✦ Age of first menstrual cycle >13 years
- ✦ History of irregular menstrual cycles before beginning athletic training
- ✦ Low body weight, or body fat percentage less than 16-18 percent
- ✦ Vegetarian diet
- ✦ Changes in body weight of more than 10 pounds in the past year
- ✦ If a runner, distance run per week >65 miles (100 km)
- ✦ If a runner, race time for 10 km run < 40 minutes
- ✦ High amounts of stress
- ✦ Inadequate diet for amount of exercise
- ✦ Disordered eating, anorexia, or bulimia
- ✦ Energy drain (taken from energy equation on page 130)
- ✦ Training seven days a week with no rest days

(The first eight items are adapted from Myburgh et al., 1992.)

Deborah lost approximately six pounds the summer between her junior and senior years in high school because of her increased cross country training. She started a low-fat, semivegetarian diet and did not eat red meat at all. She had started her menstrual periods at age 13 years and four months, a little later than her classmates. Her first periods were irregular and light in flow, occurring only about six or seven times a year; they completely stopped when she was a senior in high school. Her training had increased from 35 to 70 miles a week. Deborah had several factors that put her at increased risk for developing amenorrhea, including a rigorous training schedule with no days off, a near-vegetarian diet, weight loss because of training, and a history of irregular menstrual cycles.

WHAT TO DO IF YOU HAVE AMENORRHEA

If you miss three or more menstrual periods, run, don't walk to your doctor for a complete evaluation. As you've learned earlier in this chapter, there are many reasons why your menstrual cycle might stop, including stress, hormone disturbances such as thyroid gland problems, medical illness, and serious problems with the ovaries or brain such as cysts or even tumors. If you are sexually active, pregnancy is also a possibility. Early recognition and treatment of any of these conditions is important for a successful outcome.

Currently there is not one laboratory test or physical examination finding that tells a doctor whether or not your amenorrhea is exercise-associated. All other causes must be ruled out by a careful physical examination and laboratory tests.

See the Doctor for an Evaluation

When seeing your doctor or other clinician for an evaluation of amenorrhea, you can help the process by having some key information available. This includes a history of your training, when you started physical activity, and how much you are doing in miles or hours per week. See if you can recall how old you were when you started your period and how many menstrual cycles per year you've had. The doctor may also want to know the ages of first menstrual periods for your mother and sisters. Expect some questions about whether your period changes when you train hard and about whether your weight has changed. A sample medical history form is included in the sidebar on page 136.

Deborah's mother disagreed with the cross country team coach, who thought that amenorrhea was a normal part of Deborah's training. She insisted that Deborah see her family doctor for a full checkup. The doctor had seen Deborah before for athletic physicals and for treatment of bronchitis. She had Deborah fill out a questionnaire about her medical history, training, menstrual cycles, and diet. Deborah's diet review showed that she followed a near-vegetarian diet with a few eggs and some milk products. Her average daily caloric intake was 1,400 calories, far less than was needed to meet her resting energy needs plus the needs of training. At 5'9", Deborah thought her ideal weight was 114 pounds, 10 pounds less than her current weight of 124 pounds. Her current weight was 13 pounds less than it had been the previous year, when she was a junior in high school.

When the doctor asked about her athletic goals, Deborah said she was trying to qualify for the state championship competition. She thought she would be faster if she lost more weight. She denied using any medications, diet pills, or purging methods. She trained seven days a week, and sometimes did an extra workout on Sunday to lose weight before the mandatory weigh-ins her coach held each Monday.

The doctor asked her how she was feeling. Deborah said she had been feeling cold lately, and somewhat tired, but did not have any headaches, vision changes, increased body hair or breast discharge. She had a right hamstring injury that had bothered her for about two months. The doctor then asked Deborah's mother to leave the room while she did a medical examination. After her mother left, the doctor asked Deborah about how much stress she was feeling. Deborah said she was working out very hard, and making the sacrifices needed to make it to the state championships. She told the doctor she felt anxious if she didn't work out every day. She admitted to missing out on a social life and to feeling tired, depressed, and obsessed about her weight a lot of the time. She also said that she had never been sexually active and wasn't worried about missing her period. In fact, she was glad that her period had stopped and did not want it back.

Menstrual History—Athletic Women

Name: _____ Date: _____

Birthdate: _____ Current age: _____

1. At what age, to the nearest month, did you begin training for competition in any sport?_____

2. To the nearest month, how old were you when you had your first menstrual period? _____

3. Would you say that this age is accurate to within one month, three months, six months, one year, or not sure (choose one)?
   _____

4. In the years after your first period (menarche), indicate in the table below how many menstrual cycles you had each year, the average length of time (in days) between cycles, and whether you took oral contraceptives (birth control pills).

Age	Year after menarche	Total # of cycles	Average # of days between cycles	Number of months you took birth control pills	Number of consecutive periods missed
	1st				
	2nd				
	3rd				
	4th				
	5th				
	6th				

5. Have you ever taken birth control pills? _____
   If yes, in your lifetime how many months would you say you have taken birth control pills? _____

6. Have you ever taken anabolic steroids? _____
   If yes, in your lifetime how many months would you say you have taken anabolic steroids? _____

7. Do you take calcium supplements? _____
   If yes, what type, amount, and for how long? _____

8. Do you drink milk?_____

If yes, how many glasses a day (average)? _____

9. Do you eat yogurt? _____

   If yes, how many cups a day (average)? _____

10. Have you ever seen a doctor or nurse for a gynecological evaluation? _____

    If yes, provide date and location. _____

11. Date your most recent menstrual period began_____

12. Average number of days between your periods in the last six months_____

13. Do you have any "warnings" (e.g., weight gain, bloating, breast tenderness) before your periods start? _____

    If yes, indicate symptoms._____

14. Do you gain weight before or during your period? _____

    If yes, how much do you gain?_____

15. What are your highest and lowest weights?

    Highest weight ___ Age ___Length of time at that weight _____

    Lowest weight _____ Age _____ Length of time at that weight _____

16. Did you have regular menstrual cycles when you were at your lowest weight?_____

17. Do you try to lose weight? _____

18. Do you lose weight when training? _____

    If yes, how much weight do you lose? _____

19. What do you consider to be your ideal weight? _____

20. Do you have any questions about your health? _____

The doctor will also ask about your diet and should inquire about disordered eating practices and the amount of stress that you are under. Questions about diet and stress are a routine part of the evaluation of amenorrhea and your health in general. The doctor will also ask about symptoms related to the endocrine system, brain, and menstrual cycle. These include questions about body-hair growth, acne, discharge from the breasts, headaches, vision changes, and sexual activity. You should take in a list of any medications or herbal products you are using.

Deborah's story is common among young athletic women with amenorrhea. Have you known anyone like her? She isn't concerned about her amenorrhea. She is trying to lose weight to please a coach or in a misguided attempt to improve athletic performance. Her drastic diet and rapid weight loss during a time of training impairs performance by sacrificing lean muscle and not providing enough nutrition for her daily energy needs. She would do better to eat a higher carbohydrate diet that fulfills her energy needs (2,400 calories a day), take at least one rest day a week, and get physical therapy for her injury that won't heal.

What about Deborah's evaluation by the doctor? What can she expect? The doctor will do a physical examination that includes a gynecological examination to check the ovaries and the uterus and a Pap smear, a screening test for cancer of the cervix. If you are seeing a doctor to evaluate amenorrhea and have not had an internal gynecological examination in the past, you should let the doctor know so that any questions or concerns you have can be answered before the examination. After the doctor takes your history and does a physical examination, he or she usually has a good idea about what is causing the amenorrhea. Many physicians say that 90 percent of the diagnosis can be determined by a careful history and examination.

However, the doctor may also order X-rays and blood tests to check the functioning of your reproductive system and to check for competing hormones that come from other glands in the body, such as your thyroid or adrenal gland. The doctor will usually measure the levels of the signaling hormones LH and FSH, made in the pituitary, as well as the level of estrogen in the bloodstream. Low levels of estrogen are found in all forms of hypothalamic amenorrhea. You may also have a screening test for anemia and a test for the iron stores (ferritin) in your body to make sure you have adequate iron to make new red blood cells. If there are indications of a problem with the ovaries or the hypothalamus or pituitary gland, X-rays or an ultrasound might be requested. If you are sexually active, expect that a pregnancy test will be ordered to make sure you are not pregnant, even if you are using a reliable form of contraception. The purpose of the physician's evaluation and the tests is to make sure that you do not have another medical condition.

Answers to Common Questions About Menstrual Periods

Q. My period comes every 25 days. Is that normal?

A. Yes. Although it may be inconvenient to have a menstrual period every 25 days, it is within the normal range. The average menstrual period occurs every 23 to 38 days.

Q. Is it normal for my periods to stop when I am training?

A. It is common for a woman's periods to stop during athletic training, but it is not normal. Up to 44 percent of women training hard may have amenorrhea. If your periods stop for three months or more, you should see a physician for a full medical evaluation. Amenorrhea is a symptom of something going wrong in the body, and you need to be checked to find out what the problem is.

Q. All the other girls on my team stop having their periods when they train hard; why do I keep having mine?

A. Most likely you are still having your period because you are healthy. Your energy is in balance, you are getting adequate rest and nutrition, and you are not overtraining.

Q. Doesn't it mean I am fit when my period stops?

A. No. It means the opposite. You are most likely overtrained if your period stops. You need to have a medical evaluation to find out why your period has stopped. If all other causes are eliminated by a medical evaluation, you may have exercise-associated amenorrhea. It is a sign that you are in energy deficit and need to improve your energy balance. You are also at risk for developing osteoporosis and overuse injuries such as stress fractures.

Q. If I don't get my period for a while, it's no big deal, is it?

A. Unfortunately, it is a big deal. You are at risk for irreversible bone loss and stress fractures, and you may have difficult getting pregnant in the future.

If you have not had your period in three months or more and are not pregnant, the doctor may give you a test dose of the hormone progesterone to cause the uterus to slough its lining. If you are given progesterone in either pill or injection form, and you respond to it by bleeding, this does not mean you have a normal menstrual cycle or that your periods will start again. Progesterone is only inducing the uterine lining to bleed. Progesterone by itself does not induce your hypothalamus to start the reproductive system functioning again. Remember that progesterone is the hormone naturally made during the second half of the normal menstrual cycle. If you are not having menstrual periods, you are not making progesterone. However, you are probably making low levels of estrogen. This estrogen will develop some lining in your uterus. Taking progesterone will cause the lining in the uterus to develop and mature just as it does when you have a normal menstrual period. After you finish taking the progesterone, if there was any lining in the uterus that the progesterone caused to mature, then it will come out in a manner similar to menstrual bleeding. Sometimes it will be just like a normal period. Other times it might be brownish in color, like old blood. If you do not bleed at all in response to the progesterone, it usually means that your estrogen level is quite low, so low that you did not have any lining in the uterus.

The progesterone may need to be given every one to three months to induce bleeding. It does not correct your menstrual cycle, rather it prevents an abnormal buildup of tissue that could become precancerous if not sloughed every three to six months.

If your evaluation reveals concern about nutrition or an eating disorder, expect to be referred to a multidisciplinary team of specialists to help you solve the problems (see chapter 7). You may consult a nutritionist to make sure you are getting adequate calcium, iron, calories, protein, and other nutrients. She can help you determine your requirements for energy balance and advise you how best to meet your nutritional needs.

When you are amenorrheic, you need at least 1,500 mg of calcium a day to stay in calcium balance (see chapter 6 for more on calcium balance)—that is the maximum that the body can use. You also need enough calories to meet your daily needs for an active life. If you are in a state of chronic energy drain or are underweight or undernourished, you may need 200 to 500 calories a day above your actual daily energy requirements for several weeks or months to catch up and correct your energy deficit. If you deal with a lot of stress, don't like your body image, or have developed an eating disorder, a psychologist or other mental health practitioner can also be part of your evaluation and treatment team. These professionals can help you deal with any issues related to stress, a poor body image, depression, or disordered eating. They can also provide performance enhancement training.

Get Needed Medical Tests

You will need to be tested for a number of other conditions that may cause amenorrhea. These conditions include the following:

- ❖ Pregnancy
- ❖ Premature ovarian failure
- ❖ Ovarian tumors
- ❖ Polycystic ovary syndrome

◆ Pituitary failure

◆ Pituitary or other brain tumors

◆ Pituitary adenoma (benign growths in the pituitary gland)

◆ Eating disorders: anorexia, bulimia

◆ Thyroid disorders (either overactive or underactive)

◆ Adrenal gland disorders

◆ Problems related to the use of anabolic steroids

Before **Deborah** left the doctor's office, she was given a prescription for progesterone pills, and she scheduled an appointment with a nutritionist. It was recommended she take at least one day off a week from training and get therapy for her injury. She was given some ideas on how to increase calcium in her diet to the level needed to keep her bones strong and healthy—1,500 mg a day. A body composition measurement by skinfolds showed that her body fat was 16 percent, plus or minus 3 percent. She was at least 2 to 10 pounds underweight for her body frame and level of physical activity, so she also was advised to increase her consumption of protein and carbohydrates and to take in between 2,250 and 2,500 calories a day so that her muscles would have the fuel they needed. Deborah was diagnosed with hypothalamic amenorrhea, and she certainly had an energy imbalance.

When Deborah heard this diagnosis, she still didn't believe anything was wrong. She was glad not to have her period, and she felt that she was training right. She did not like the advice to rest, change her diet, and eat more. When she went back to see the doctor, she had actually lost a half-pound since her previous visit. The doctor was worried about her inability to make changes and feared that Deborah was in the early stages of anorexia. She referred Deborah to a sport psychologist to help in her evaluation and treatment. The doctor was also concerned that Deborah might have osteoporosis, another component of the female athlete triad. The doctor told Deborah that she might have low bone mass and recommended a bone density test.

Consequences of Amenorrhea

For many years, it was felt that there were no immediate nor future health problems for women with amenorrhea. Today we know that there are several serious consequences. These include osteoporosis and infertility. Recall what happens to women after menopause, when they are not producing female hormones or are producing very low levels. Similar things happen to young women who have amenorrhea—their ovaries do not produce any eggs or hormones. In menopausal women, the low levels of hormones, especially estrogen, can lead to a rapid loss of bone mineral (osteoporosis), increased risk of heart disease, hot flashes, dry skin and vaginal tissue, diminished sexual desire, and memory loss. Replacing the ovarian hormones can treat these problems in menopausal women, but what about in women with hypothalamic amenorrhea?

Although medical research has only just begun to evaluate the short- and long-term consequences of amenorrhea in athletes, we have learned some lessons from the study of menopausal women. The situation of an athlete with amenorrhea is similar to that of a woman after menopause. Both have low levels of estrogen. We know now that young women do get osteoporosis. We don't have much information about increased risk of heart disease or memory problems. There is some indirect evidence that being estrogen deficient at a young age can increase the risk for scoliosis (curvature of the spine) and athletic injuries, including stress fractures (see figure 5.2).

Osteoporosis

The groundbreaking studies of Dr. Barbara Drinkwater and others in the early 1980s linked amenorrhea to dangerously thin bones in athletes. Women in their 20s who had amenorrhea were found to have the bone density of women in their 50s and even 70s. This bone loss has been called old bones in young women. The osteoporosis caused by low estrogen levels in young women with amenorrhea is the third part of the female athlete triad. In fact, a woman's bone density can be predicted by reviewing her menstrual history. The fewer menstrual cycles, the lower her bone density. See chapter 6 for more information about osteoporosis.

Difficulty Getting Pregnant

One concern for many women with amenorrhea women is their future ability to have children. If you aren't having periods, can you get pregnant? Well, the answer is both yes and no. What, you say? How can you get pregnant if you are not having your period?! Remember that in the human menstrual cycle, a woman releases an egg before she menstruates. Thus, if a woman is recovering from amenorrhea, she will ovulate before she starts menstruating again. If she is sexually active and is not using contraception, that egg can be fertilized and can result in pregnancy without her ever having a period. Olympic marathoner Ingrid Kristiansen and others have become pregnant this way. When Kristiansen took some time off from training, her energy balance returned to normal, and she ovulated. It is important to know that if you have amenorrhea and are sexually active, there is a chance you can get pregnant. If you don't want to be pregnant, make sure you use a reliable form of contraception.

Women who do not correct their energy imbalance or who have a medical condition causing amenorrhea are unable to get pregnant until the cause of their amenorrhea is reversed. The longer a woman has amenorrhea, especially because of an energy imbalance, the more difficult it may be to reverse and the less likely it is that she can get pregnant. In those cases, if a woman wants to become pregnant, she should first have the cause of her amenorrhea diagnosed and treated. She may need to see a fertility specialist for hormonal treatments that will induce ovulation.

GETTING BETTER

Treatment of amenorrhea and oligomenorrhea depends on first determining the cause and then taking action to correct it. If, as in Rowena's case, the amenorrhea is due to exercise-related energy drain and overtraining, then correcting the energy imbalance will likely reverse it. If the amenorrhea is part of the female athlete triad, then it is important that the full spectrum of the triad disorders be evaluated and treated. If recognized and treated early, the serious consequences of eating disorders can be avoided. If there are signs of disordered eating and body image distortion, then a key part of treatment is dealing with those issues with a mental health professional. Deborah is an example of a young woman with amenorrhea who has some features of disordered eating. She initially does not seem able or willing to make the changes necessary to correct her amenorrhea by improved nutrition, weight gain, and modified training. She is typical of a woman with the female athlete triad.

Rowena, the former college gymnast with irregular menstrual periods (see page 112), was trying to get pregnant. At age 27, she and her husband had been trying to start a family for a year and a half. She only had two or three menstrual cycles a year. She tried to check her basal body temperature and use home kits to see if she was ovulating, but they never seemed to show ovulation. She was watching her weight as she had always done, sticking to the low-fat, vegetarian diet that she had used to keep thin since her days as a gymnast. She was still at her college competition weight. She taught aerobics five nights a week and usually went for long bike rides on the weekends. Finally, after trying to get pregnant for almost two years, she went to see a fertility specialist. After examining her and doing blood tests as well as checking her husband's sperm count, the doctor told Rowena that she was not ovulating regularly. He felt the cause was her low body weight and very active lifestyle. He suggested that she gain 5 to 10 pounds and cut back on the exercise so that she had at least two days off a week. He also told her that fertility drugs were an option if she did not start ovulating in six months, and he advised her to get a bone density test.

Rowena did not want to gain weight. She had been trying to stay slim so as to avoid gaining too much weight during her anticipated pregnancy. The forces that had always driven her to diet and work out were still keeping her underweight, with inadequate energy to start up her reproductive system. However, faced with the prospect of either not having a family or taking fertility drugs, Rowena found that her focus changed. It no longer mattered so much to her what she weighed or whether she could still fit into a size four. She wanted a family. With her husband's encouragement, she started eating more and sometimes even had dessert. She cut down on teaching aerobics. Her bone density test came out slightly lower than normal, and she added more dairy products and other sources of calcium to her diet to ensure that she was getting 1,500 mg of calcium a day. About six months after these changes, her doctor found that she was ovulating naturally. She started to have monthly periods, and three months later she was pregnant.

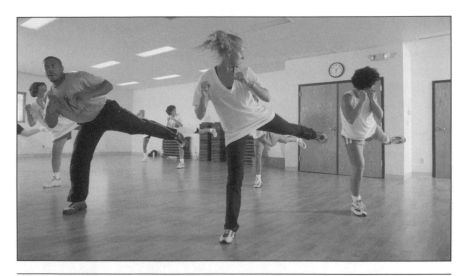

By correcting an energy imbalance—eating a nutritious diet that fuels the body and replaces energy spent by exercise—you can often regain normal menstrual periods.

Deborah met with the sport psychologist and also had a bone density test done on her hips and lower spine. The psychologist found that Deborah had a high drive for thinness and was mistakenly viewing herself as fat. The bone density test showed that Deborah had lost more than 10 percent of her bone mass and was at risk for osteoporosis. Deborah's doctor saw her in a follow-up visit and again urged her to increase her nutrition to ensure 1,500 mg of calcium a day in her diet, to get 2,400 calories a day, to take one day a week off from running, and to gain some weight.

Deborah's running times and performance had not improved in spite of her added training. The doctor told her that she was running on empty and was too thin to win. Deborah did not believe her and felt that she was not improving in her races because of the time the medical tests were taking away from her running. Deborah still was focused on making the state championship competition. She did not want to make any changes until after the qualifying meet. Given Deborah's reluctance to make some changes in her diet and lifestyle, the doctor requested a family conference to review all the findings and recommendations.

Take In More Calcium

Every woman who experiences amenorrhea needs to make sure that she gets 1,500 mg of calcium a day to stay in calcium balance. If you do not get this amount, you are likely to lose more bone mass from your skeleton. Many people think that by taking in more calcium, you are increasing your bone mass. Not true. Calcium is the raw material needed to build bone. You also need estrogen (or testosterone, if you are a man) to carry the calcium to the bone. Even if you take in 1,500 mg of calcium or more a day, you will not build bone unless you correct the hormone deficiency of amenorrhea and restore normal levels of estrogen and other female hormones. Getting the required amount of calcium does not build bone; it just keeps the proper amount available to the body. A higher intake of calcium (above 1,500 mg) does not help you build more bone; it is just excreted in the urine. The best sources of calcium are foods. Food sources are better than supplement sources, because the body more easily absorbs them. But if you find it difficult to get enough calcium from food sources, you can use calcium supplements. (See chapter 6 for more on calcium requirements.)

Balance Your Training

Some athletic women with amenorrhea do not have the psychological aspects of disordered eating, but they find themselves inadvertently in an energy deficit because they train so hard. This is most likely to occur in women training for endurance-type events. It is likely that their exercise-associated amenorrhea is a sign of overtraining. There is a fine line between adequate training and overtraining. When a woman is overtraining, her performance declines and injuries occur. Coaches and athletes must recognize and correct this problem if they want to be successful.

Wise coaches and athletes recognize that amenorrhea is an early marker for overtraining, not a sign that the training is hard enough. Athletic women who do not have the body image distortion and the psychological problems related to disordered eating can make a few lifestyle changes, such as correcting their energy deficit by increasing their food intake, resting, and reducing training, to correct the overtraining.

The first evidence that minor lifestyle changes would help reverse exercise-associated amenorrhea came from studies of athletic women with amenorrhea who were told about their low bone mass. The women were worried about their low bone mass and modified their training.

In some cases they had become injured and were forced to take time off from training and competition. Most women in the studies decreased training for two to four months, and gained between two and seven pounds. Their menstruation resumed, and later measurements showed that their bone density had increased, although it did not completely return to normal.

On the basis of these early studies, other investigators have done more controlled studies on athletic women. In one recent study, cross country runners at a junior college were found to be in energy drain, and they followed advice to correct their energy imbalances. When these athletes improved their nutrition by an average of just 350 calories a day and took one day off a week from training, their running times improved and, in some cases, their hormone imbalances reversed! This study showed that athletic women who make even minor lifestyle changes can improve their performance.

Adjust Your Diet

Lifestyle changes to correct your energy imbalance should be individualized for you by a doctor or nutritionist (see page 130 of this chapter to calculate your energy needs). Most women need to add about 250 to 350 calories a day and ensure that they get 1,500 mg of calcium in order to stay in balance. An easy way to do both is to add calcium-rich foods such as calcium-fortified orange juice, sport bars, yogurt, nonfat milk, or tofu to the diet (see also chapter 6). The best way to add calories and improve your performance is to take in the additional 200 to 400 calories provided by a carbohydrate-rich food or drink source in the 30 to 90 minutes after you exercise. Adding carbohydrate at this time replenishes the glycogen stores in the muscles in the most efficient manner. These added calories will fuel your performance the next day. If you wait longer than two hours, you may not store the calories as fuel for your muscles. Choose sport drinks, fruit juice, sport bars, bagels, Fig Newtons, fruit, or a sandwich to meet your energy needs and power up your muscles. In addition to making dietary changes, some women may need to gain two to seven pounds if they have a long history of energy drain or if their symptoms of overtraining were associated with weight loss.

Add More Rest

Correcting an energy deficit and resuming menstruation can also involve taking some time off from training. Most professional athletes do not train seven days a week, and if they do, they are making a mistake. Even God took one day off! At least one rest day a week should be built into a training schedule. Athletes should take one day off after tough competitions, and they should vary their training schedules, doing heavy workouts on some days and light workouts on other days. If an athlete makes all of the recommended lifestyle changes, it usually takes three to six months for her menstrual periods to resume normally.

Having a normal menstrual cycle gives you the benefits of all the ovarian hormones you are meant to have. These hormones play important roles in the growth and development of your musculoskeletal system and in cardiovascular health, sexuality, and immunity. Women are meant to have monthly menstrual cycles, and they need the ovarian hormones to build their peak bone mass. Getting your menstrual cycle back to normal is a clear indicator that a previous underlying energy imbalance is corrected.

Replace Missing Hormones

Many women find it difficult to correct energy imbalances, particularly during a competitive season. Some women have had amenorrhea for several years before seeking medical advice and already have a serious loss of bone mineral density. Others have had stress fractures and do not want to have more. What can be done for an active woman who needs the immediate protection of balanced hormones but is unable to make the lifestyle changes necessary to restore her menstrual cycle? For certain women with amenorrhea, the missing hormones may need to be replaced, although these women should still take action to correct their energy imbalances and take a rest day, which will improve their performance. The easiest way to replace missing hormones is to take birth control pills. They provide both estrogen and progesterone in doses that have been shown to prevent bone loss, provide contraception, and regulate menstrual bleeding. This may be the first choice of treatment for a woman who also wants to use the pill for contraception. But a woman does not need to be sexually active to benefit from this type of hormone replacement. There are several known benefits to the pill—among them, reduction in acne and decreased risk of ovarian and endometrial (uterine lining) cancer—in addition to their protective effect on the bones.

Some women may not like taking birth control pills because of concerns over weight gain or other side effects, or decreased performance. To date, there is no reliable evidence that birth control pills decrease athletic performance in women. The average weight gain is usually less than two pounds. There are over 20 different types of birth control pills, and if a woman elects to try this course of therapy, she can work with her clinician to find a pill that doesn't give her unwanted side effects such as breast enlargement or weight gain.

Remember, taking birth control pills or any other form of hormone replacement does not correct the underlying cause of amenorrhea. It does not restore fertility. The goal of this treatment is to replace some of the hormones made by the ovaries. By replacing the missing hormones, a woman is also acting to slow down bone loss. As previously mentioned, women who use birth control pills to help treat their amenorrhea also need to make the lifestyle changes in diet and training that will correct their energy imbalances and restore regular menstrual periods. In my practice, if a woman cannot reverse her amenorrhea with lifestyle changes in three to six months, then we will try hormone replacement while continuing the diet, rest, and recovery of her energy balance. When she has been in an energy balanced state for two to six months, I then suggest that she stop the oral contraceptives and see if her normal menstruation resumes.

Deborah's mother came in for a family conference with the doctor and the nutritionist. She was told that Deborah was in an energy deficient state and that as a result her body was conserving energy by stopping her menstrual cycles. Since her menstrual cycles had stopped, she did not have the estrogen needed to put calcium into her bones, and she already showed a loss of bone mass. She was at risk for a stress fracture. Deborah's mother was concerned, and she agreed to a plan to add calcium-rich foods to Deborah's diet. Together, she and Deborah would talk to the coach. With the doctor and nutritionist, they looked at the printout of Deborah's bone density test. Somehow, seeing in print that her bones were thin really shocked Deborah. Her grandmother had osteoporosis, and she definitely did not want to get that. Deborah also was constantly tired and stressed out from training, always watching her weight, and not eating normally. Her running times were not improving, and she admitted to icing her hamstring every day. Faced with all the evidence, she finally agreed to make some changes in her diet, modify her training, and take a calcium supplement. She also went to see a physical therapist to help with her hamstring injury and agreed to continue seeing the psychologist.

(continued)

When Deborah returned for follow-up eight weeks later, she had gained two pounds and had qualified for state championships. She did not want to take birth control pills. Instead, with the consent of her doctor, she decided to see if lifestyle changes would help her period come back normally in three to four months. In the next few weeks, she added more calcium-rich foods to her diet, continued to take a day off from training each week and she gained a few more pounds. Her hamstring injury improved, and two months later her menstrual cycle returned. Although she did not welcome its return, she had heard enough from her advisors and her mother that she now saw her period as a normal part of a healthy life. She felt better and had more energy even though she wasn't the thinnest girl on the team. She was running better than ever, producing her best times, and she had a good chance for a college scholarship.

WHAT DEBORAH'S, DIANE'S, AND ROWENA'S EXPERIENCES TEACH US

Deborah, Diane, and Rowena all experienced changes in their menstrual cycles associated with their exercise and diet. While these changes are common in athletic women, menstrual changes cannot be blamed solely on exercise. Each woman had to have a medical workup to determine the cause of these changes, to rule out causes such as hormone imbalance, brain tumor, or even pregnancy. It has only recently been discovered that amenorrhea and delayed menarche can have negative consequences on performance and bone health.

Starting puberty late is not normal.

Diane, the young gymnast, had not started her periods by age 14. Her parents were concerned enough to get her medically evaluated. Her doctor recommended some nutritional changes and ran some tests to determine the cause. Although it has been observed that athletes have a later age of menarche, other serious medical problems must be ruled out before deciding that the delay is due to exercise. Additionally, delayed menarche has been associated with scoliosis and stress fractures.

Action to take: If you do not begin puberty (breast development) by age 12 or 13, or do not start your periods by age 16, you need to see a doctor for a complete checkup to determine the cause of your delayed puberty.

Stopping your periods is not a sign of fitness.

By now you should know amenorrhea is a sign of an underlying medical problem that needs a thorough evaluation. Deborah's coach and teammates mistakenly viewed amenorrhea as a marker of exceptional training. However, in reality it is a marker of overtraining and energy drain. They, like many others, did not understand the full implications for their performance and health.

Action to take: If you experience a disruption or change in your menstruation, you should seek medical care. Deborah's mother disagreed with the cross country team coach and insisted Deborah get a full workup. This helped Deborah get the care she needed and avoid serious long-term consequences like osteoporosis (see chapter 6). The medical evaluation should include a full history, physical, and blood tests. If your doctor says it is a normal for athletic women to not have their periods, show her this book! Or get another opinion. See chapter 7 for guidelines on how to choose an appropriate physician.

Amenorrhea is a sign of overtraining.

Deborah increased her training dramatically over the summer for the fall cross country season. She developed fatigue, staleness, a hamstring injury, and amenorrhea. Deborah was found to have an energy deficit of 1000 calories a day and was training seven days a week, sometimes twice on Sunday. After other causes of amenorrhea were ruled out by her doctor, her symptoms were determined to be a result of overtraining and inadequate diet.

Action to take: If you are training intensely, monitor yourself for overtraining by knowing the symptoms (see page 127) and keeping a training log (see page 128). You can prevent overtraining by computing your energy equation (see page 130) and making sure you meet your dietary needs. Also, vary your hard and easy days and get at least one rest day a week to consolidate the gains from your training.

If your periods stop, or if you have fewer than six a year, you need more calcium in your diet.

Deborah, the cross country runner, was found to have low bone mass due to her amenorrhea. Once a woman's periods stop, whether it be as a young woman or after menopause, she starts to lose bone mass which may never be replaced.

Action to take: Women without regular menstrual periods need 1500 mg of calcium a day to stay in calcium balance. See chapter 6 for more information on how you can meet this daily requirement. It is important to realize that getting this much calcium does not help you build bone or prevent bone loss. It only ensures that your bones get their minimum daily requirement and keeps your body from removing calcium from your bones. To build bone or prevent bone loss, your menstrual cycles need to return to normal, or you need to take replacement hormones.

Stopping your periods means it can be difficult to get pregnant.

Rowena tried to get pregnant for two years when she was 27 years old. She was a former gymnast and aerobics instructor and never had regular periods. Her doctors considered giving her fertility drugs, however she was able to make lifestyle changes and eventually got pregnant naturally.

Action to take: See a doctor to determine the cause of your irregular periods and get the correct treatment. If the causes of irregular menstruation are not reversed, you may not ovulate regularly and will find it difficult to get pregnant.

Even if your periods have stopped, it is possible to get pregnant.

Recall that in the normal menstrual cycle a woman produces an egg before she menstruates. Although it is not common, sexually active athletes with amenorrhea have unknowingly resumed ovulation and gotten pregnant without resuming menstruation. For several months, they were unaware of their condition because they believed their amenorrhea was a result of their exercise.

Action to take: If you experience amenorrhea and are sexually active, continue to use an effective form of contraception if you do not want to become pregnant.

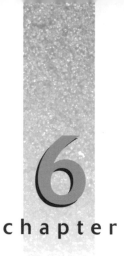

6

c h a p t e r

Old Bones in
Young Women:
Osteoporosis

Bones are the hidden heroes of our bodies. They are the framework for our leaps and bounds, the structure for our sitting and running, and the foundation for working and playing. It may surprise you to know that bones are in a constant state of growth and remodeling. Unseen and unfelt, our bones are growing daily, and they reach maximum strength when we are approximately 30 years old. Anything that goes wrong during these 30 years of growth may cause our bones to be weaker than they should be. Without strong bones, we do not have the support to run, jump, straighten, turn, or even breathe right. With injured bones, we are in pain and off balance. We need to fight any condition that attacks the integrity of our bones if we are to maintain our vigor. Fortunately, one of the most common conditions that affect bones—loss of bone density, or osteoporosis—is preventable.

153

Leah, whom we met in chapter 1, was the best runner on her high school track team. However, when she went to college, she found she was only average. She followed the lead of her teammates in dieting to be lean and mean and lost 10 pounds her first semester. Her running times did not improve much. Her track workouts were tougher than in high school, and she started having lower-leg pain. The pain was gone in the mornings but got worse during the day and was really bad after practices. She saw the team doctor, who ordered a bone scan test. She was found to have two stress fractures in her left lower-leg. Her freshman track season was gone! Her doctor told her it would take at least six weeks of rest and limited activity to heal the stress fractures.

Most of you probably think osteoporosis only affects your grand-mothers or older women, but it can and does seriously change the lives of young, active women like Leah. Osteoporosis starts when bone mass or density is lost, causing the bone to become weak. This weakness can result in three different types of fractures; stress, crush, and complete fractures. When they are in this weakened state, the bones are susceptible to cracks just from everyday activities or work-outs! Stress fractures are different from regular, complete bone frac-tures that result from a sudden, explosive impact. Stress fractures are caused by repeated stress over time that causes a crack in the architecture of the bone. If the bone is weakened by osteoporosis, stress fractures are more likely to occur.

Stress fractures are common and disabling injuries that can hap-pen to any active woman, whether she is just starting an exercise program or is training intensively for competition. As we have dis-cussed throughout this book, the development of osteoporosis in active women under age 50 has been linked to the other two triad conditions of disordered eating and amenorrhea. Disordered eating practices hinder the nutritional intake necessary for maintaining bone health. They also contribute to amenorrhea, which leads to low es-trogen and impaired bone development. Unfortunately, osteoporo-sis may advance undetected for years before the condition is discov-ered after a fracture. If you don't take the necessary steps to prevent losing bone mass as a young, active woman, you increase your risk of losing bone density that you can't get back and developing weakened bones as you get older.

Fortunately, you can do a great deal to prevent losing bone mass and to protect your bones from becoming brittle. The time to prevent osteoporosis is before age 30, when your bone mass is being developed. Then you must continue to do the right things for your bones as you get older. In this chapter we review what osteoporosis is as well as how you can prevent it. In addition, we discuss who is at risk and how stress fractures develop. We also explain how bone develops and the critical roles calcium, estrogen, and exercise play in bone development and maintenance. You'll learn how to make sure you provide your body with the calcium, estrogen levels, and exercise you need at all stages of your life to ensure healthy bones. You'll also find out what to do if you do have a stress fracture or low bone density and how to treat it.

WHAT IS OSTEOPOROSIS?

Osteoporosis comes from the Greek *osteo,* meaning bones, and *porosis*, meaning porous. Think of a sponge with its holes and pores. If the sponge holes enlarged and the sponge mesh shrank, then the sponge would look like osteoporotic bone (see figure 6.1a). Not the type you'd want to be jumping out of airplanes with! Or doing step aerobics or jogging down the street with, for that matter. Osteoporotic bone contains more holes and less solid mineral than normal bone (see figure 6.1b). It is also brittle, weak, and more likely to break or fracture. Swiss cheese for bone? No way! Not if you want to stay healthy and fit.

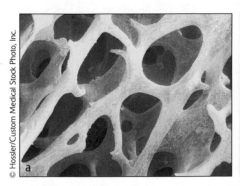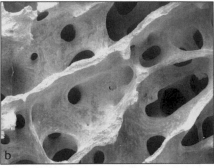

© Hossler/Custom Medical Stock Photo, Inc.

Figure 6.1 Detatiled veiw of (a) osteoporotic and (b) normal bone.

WHO IS AT RISK?

Would it surprise you to learn that no one really knows how big the problem of osteoporosis is for young women? The first studies were done on women after menopause. We know that 25 million Americans over 60 and 75 million people worldwide over 60 have osteoporosis. Eighty percent are postmenopausal women.

Osteoporosis is more often diagnosed in postmenopausal women because the outward signs of the condition are more apparent. Why is it that some older women appear hunched over and cannot straighten their backs? Do you know anyone, perhaps in your family, who has this hunched-over appearance, commonly referred to as dowager's hump (see figure 6.2a)? When young women are asked why they think some older women look this way, they often say it is because the women are too tired or too weak. However, the real reason for this deforming posture is that the bones in these women's spines have become weak and broken. They break in a wedge-shaped crush fracture that causes the bones to bend forward (figure 6.2b). Such crush fractures occur with almost no injury at all. A woman with this problem cannot stand up straight because her spine is permanently bent due to these osteoporotic fractures. Not only can she not stand up straight, she also cannot take a full breath of air, and her stomach and other organs in the abdomen are compressed on each other.

Does it seem like this could never happen to you? Unfortunately, it can. There are numerous recorded cases of the same spinal crush fractures in young women who have lost bone because of anorexia and amenorrhea.

Risk Profile Questionnaire

General Profile

Are you

   __ female?   (2 points)

   __ Caucasian or Asian?   (2 points)

   __ descended from ancestors born in Northern Europe, The British Isles, China, or Japan?   (2points)

Do you

   __ have a small build (size 8 dress or less)?

                                                   (2 points)

__ have light hair, a fair complexion, or freckles? (2 points)

__ consume fewer than two milk products per day? (2 points)

__ exercise less than 30 minutes per day or less
than 5 miles per week of brisk walking? (2 points)

__ drink five or more cups of coffee, tea, and/or
soda daily? (2 points)

__ drink three or more alcoholic beverages daily? (7 points)

__ smoke two or more packs of cigarettes per week? (7 points)

Medical History

Are you

__ postmenopausal? (2 points)

__ If yes, did you experience menopause before
age 40? (10 points)

Do you have

__ a medical history of epilepsy, rheumatoid
arthritis, liver disease, juvenile diabetes, or
thyroid problems? (2 points)

__ a history of osteoporosis in your family? (2 points)

__ scoliosis? (7 points)

Have you

__ ever breastfed? (2 points)

__ ever fractured your wrist, hip, or spine? (2 points)

__ ever taken corticosteroids for at least one year? (10 points)

__ experienced the absense of your menstrual
cycle for more than one year (excluding
menopause)? (10 points)

Scoring: For each item checked, add the number of points to the
right of that item.

17 points or more = high risk

6 to 16 points = moderate risk

8 points or less = low risk

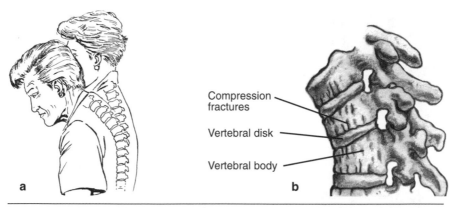

Figure 6.2 Dowager's hump (a) results from compression fractures of the bones (b).

By its very nature, osteoporosis is a silent disease in most younger women. It cannot be detected by looking at someone or by asking a few questions. Rather, it is typically diagnosed only when a fracture occurs or when there is an abnormally low measurement of bone density. (We describe how bone density is measured on page 190.) Most young women do not have bone density measurements done routinely. Until recently, it was not standard care to check a young woman with a fracture for osteoporosis. However, since the links have been made among

Alexandra is 26 years old and has just started a new job and a new exercise program. She began walking with two friends and found she enjoyed the companionship and exercising outside. However, she wanted more of a challenge. Along with her friends, she joined the local gym and signed up for an aerobics class similar to one that she had taken a few years before. She used her walking shoes for the class and noticed a pain in the middle of her foot after the first two weeks of classes. She tried icing it before and after the class and using an ace wrap around her foot. The pain went away in the mornings but got worse if she went to aerobics or climbed a lot of stairs. By the sixth week she was in so much pain she was limping after class. She saw her primary care doctor, who took an X-ray and told her she had a stress fracture in a metatarsal bone of her foot. The doctor told her to stop aerobics and start bicycling or swimming to keep fit instead, and to increase the calcium in her diet to make sure she got 1,500 mg a day.

osteoporosis, amenorrhea, and disordered eating in athletic women, many more young women are now being evaluated for low bone mass.

Osteoporosis also makes itself apparent as a complete fracture. In older women, the most common fractures are of the hip. Fully one-third to one-half of women who break their hips never return to an independent lifestyle. Younger women also have been reported to break the bones of the hips and upper legs. Most of the fractures recorded in young women are the incomplete breaks known as stress fractures.

HOW ARE STRESS FRACTURES RELATED TO OSTEOPOROSIS?

Leah and Alexandra are two women who took two very different routes to getting a stress fracture. Leah was training right at the edge of her maximum ability, and a sudden increase in training led to her stress fractures. Alexandra, on the other hand, was just starting a health and fitness program. With such different training regimens and goals, why did both of these women get stress fractures? First, let's review what a stress fracture is. Then it may become clear why Leah and Alexandra fractured.

What does a stress fracture look like up close and personal? If you could look inside the bone with a microscope, you would see an incomplete break across part of the bone. These breaks occur at the areas of bone remodeling, the constant, lifelong urban renewal project going on in your bones so that they can withstand the forces of your physical activity. In fact, physical activity spurs the building of bone, particularly weight-bearing activities such as running and muscle-building activities like weight lifting. However, when your bone has too much stress too soon, something has to give. If the bones don't get the nutrients they need to build and repair themselves, then the stress of such weight-bearing activities will be too much. Most stress fractures occur in the bones of the lower legs and feet, because these are the areas of the body that take the most strain from bearing weight (see figure 6.3). However, stress fractures have also been reported in the arms and ribs of rowers, weight lifters, and tennis and softball players due to the extreme muscular forces that affect their upper bodies.

The traditional thinking about stress fractures is that they are over-use injuries from weight-bearing or muscular exercise. For example, women frequently develop stress fractures after doing too much mileage in a worn-out pair of shoes or participating in an aerobics class that is too hard for their level of muscular fitness. You can even get a stress fracture from too much walking before your body has adapted to it.

Stress fractures are also common in male and female soldiers starting basic training, who march for long distances.

However, now you know that stress fractures are related to other health concerns that decrease fitness and athletic performance—specifically amenorrhea and eating disorders. Groundbreaking research done in the 1980s by Dr. Barbara Drinkwater and others found that stress fractures occurred in women runners with amenorrhea and low bone mass. We know that bone loss due to the disorders of the female athlete triad contributes to stress fractures. You are setting yourself up for a stress fracture if you are exercising but not getting enough calcium to your bones or not producing enough estrogen to help build bone.

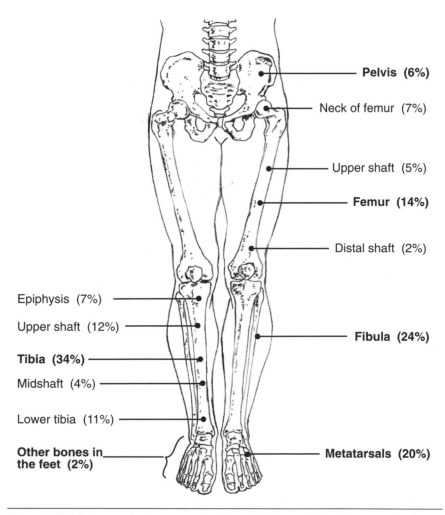

Figure 6.3 Most stress fractures occur in the pelvis, legs, and feet, but upper body stress fractures are also possible.

BONE DEVELOPMENT:
HOW YOUR SKELETON GROWS

Although you don't see or feel it happening, the skeleton is constantly changing and remodeling itself to be strongest where you place the most load in your training and in your daily life. If you are running, your bone remodeling units will increase bone in your feet and lower legs. If you are a right-handed tennis player, the muscles and bones of your entire right arm will hypertrophy (get bigger).

How does bone do it? Bone is made up of small remodeling units. There are two principal types of cells: those that build bone—called osteoblasts—and those that break down bone—called osteoclasts. Their functions are normally linked to achieve a balance between bone breaking down and building up. Bone loss results when the resorption of bone is no longer linked to bone formation; thus more bone is removed than is built up.

Bone Types: Cortical and Trabecular

Our skeletons have two types of bone in them. One type is called compact, or cortical, bone. It is the bone in the central shafts of our arms and legs, and it makes up about 80 percent of the total skeleton. This type of bone undergoes remodeling at a slower rate than the second type of bone, known as trabecular bone. Trabecular bone is located in the spine and at the ends of the long bones in the wrist and hip areas. It is the type of bone that is affected by estrogen deficiency. And because it has a higher rate of remodeling, trabecular bone is the most sensitive indicator of bone loss. Therefore, the tests that measure bone density usually measure the trabecular bones, specifically those in the lower spine and the hip (see page 190 of this chapter for more information on bone density measurements).

Achieving Peak Bone Mass

Your bones grow every day of your life (see figure 6.4). Looking at the graph, notice what happens during the years of puberty (ages 12 to 17 for girls). This is the time of the greatest rate of bone growth, when you may gain as much as 25 percent of your total bone mass. It is a critically important time to ensure that you build as much bone as possible. After you go through puberty and reach your adult height, you have about 70 percent of your genetically determined maximum bone mass. After that time, until about age 25 to 35, you are not making longer or taller bones, but rather denser and stronger bones

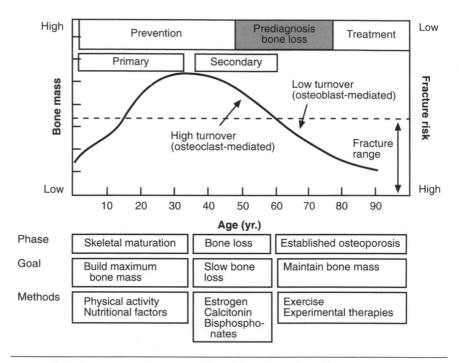

Figure 6.4 The process of bone growth and loss throughout life.

Reprinted from *American Journal of Medicine* 91 (5B) R.D. Wasnich, "Bone mass measurements in diagnosis and assessment of therapy," 54S-58S, Copyright © 1991, with permission from Excerpta Medica, Inc.

through skeletal consolidation—continuing to put deposits in your bone bank. After age 35, bone mass begins to decline as part of the aging process. Around the age of 50, the average age of menopause, it begins to decline rapidly due to the absence of female hormones.

Maximum or peak bone mass refers to the genetically determined highest amount of bone mineral that you should have in your skeleton. Peak bone mass reflects your genetic potential and also the sum of everything, good or bad, that happens to your bones during puberty and early adulthood. If anything—like a nutritional deficiency, lack of weight-bearing exercise, or an illness that requires extensive bed rest—happens during those years to impair the development of bone, you are likely to never reach your peak bone mass. From what researchers have learned about women with the female athlete triad, the bone loss is irreplaceable. If you do not reach your peak bone mass, you are heading toward osteoporosis. If you have 70 percent or less of the peak bone mass for your given age, then your bone is very weak and is likely to fracture with little trauma.

Thus, a bone mineral density that is 70 percent of the peak bone mass makes for bone that is at the fracture threshold, a dangerous place to be at any time of life.

What can you do to ensure that you reach your peak bone mass? It's not too hard. There are three things that are most important.

1. Start your menstrual periods by age 14 or earlier and have regular menstrual periods so that you know the female hormone levels within your body are adequate. See chapter 5 for more information.

2. Get your daily dose of calcium, the bone-building mineral (see table 6.1 to see how much you need). Adequate nutrition with sufficient calcium and other minerals for bone growth is very important. Growing children need up to 1,200 to 1,500 mg of calcium a day to have adequate minerals to build the growing skeleton, the same as adult women.

3. Make sure you exercise regularly. Particularly when you are growing taller during puberty, exercise induces your bones to grow stronger. The type of exercise that is most important is the type that loads the bone with more body weight than happens when you are just walking. Consider adding gymnastics activities such as jumping and tumbling, high-impact aerobics, or jumping rope to your exercise routine. Doing some weight lifting two or three times a week can also help build bone density by strengthening the muscles around the bones.

From what you know about the female athlete triad, you can probably list a few factors that can delay or limit the growth of the skeleton. Delayed menarche (see chapter 5), episodes of amenorrhea, deficient nutrition, and eating disorders all have been linked to impaired bone mineralization at the critical time of skeletal growth. Other factors that might also decrease your skeleton's growth include taking certain medications (especially corticosteroids such as prednisone, when taken for three months or longer, and antiseizure medications), smoking, abusing alcohol, and lacking other vitamins and minerals.

Role of Calcium

So what is the big deal about calcium? Calcium is a threshold nutrient for bone. It needs to be supplied to the cells that build the skeleton (the osteoblasts) so that they can use it like bricks and mortar to build the bone's framework. The osteoblasts mix calcium with phosphorus

Table 6.1
Daily Calcium Needs by Age

Age range	Needs (mg a day)	Equivalent in number of dairy servings
1 to 3	500	2 servings
3 to 8	800	3 servings
8 to 24	1,200 to 1,500	4 servings
24 to 50	1,000	3 servings
51 and older	1,200	4–5 servings
Estrogen deficient	1,500	4–5 servings

Recommendations based on the NIH Consensus Conference on Optimal Calcium Intake (June, 1994) and National Academy of Sciences–National Research Council Dietary Reference Intakes (November, 1997).

into a mineral complex. If you take in less calcium than is needed to do the job, then they do not have the building blocks for strong enough bones. The extremes of calcium deprivation are seen in malnourished children whose bones do not develop correctly. They are bow-legged and have a condition known as rickets, in which the bones are softer than normal.

Ninety-eight percent of the body's calcium is stored in the skeleton and teeth. The remaining 2 percent is found in the body fluids, where it regulates nerve transmission, blood clotting, and muscle contraction. With such major roles to play in the body, calcium must be constantly available, especially if you wish to reach your best athletic performance without injury. Your body must keep normal levels in the bloodstream even when you are not replenishing your body's supply by calcium intake. Thus, if your calcium intake is less than your daily needs, the body will rob the skeleton of calcium to keep the level in the bloodstream normal. It is as though the bones are banks where calcium can be deposited and withdrawn as needed. If your diet chronically lacks calcium, you will pay the price—perhaps not today, but years from now—in weakening of the bones.

The body makes a number of substances that regulate calcium levels in the blood. These include vitamin D, parathyroid hormone, estrogen, progesterone, testosterone, calcitonin, and thyroid hormone. Each of these substances acts to either increase calcium in the bloodstream, help calcium absorption, or remove calcium from the bones.

True or False?

A blood test can tell you if you have enough calcium.
False. There is only a small amount, less than 2 percent, of total body calcium in the bloodstream. Even with a low intake of calcium, the blood level of calcium is kept normal by the calcium-regulating hormones. Thus, you cannot tell if you are calcium deficient on the basis of the blood test. In some situations, if you are taking certain medications or have bulimia or anorexia, it is possible to force the level of calcium in your bloodstream below normal. If the calcium level in your bloodstream goes too low, you will experience serious medical problems, such as muscle cramps, spasms, prolonged muscle contractions, and irregular or skipped heartbeats.

Calcium Pluses and Minuses

Did your mom make you drink milk when you were growing up? If she did, you can thank her for helping you prevent osteoporosis. It is clear that bone development is greatest during childhood and puberty. You can maximize bone development by meeting or exceeding your daily calcium needs with foods such as milk, other dairy products, calcium-fortified orange juice, broccoli, and tofu. Recall that young girls going through puberty need 1,200 to 1,500 mg a day to reach their potential bone mass. And what if you or your friends do not get this high amount of calcium intake between ages 12 and 14? One recent study showed that even with a calcium intake of 1,200 mg a day, girls aged 12 to 14 years reached only 65 percent of their age-adjusted peak bone mass compared to girls who got 1,500 mg a day. Realistically, how many girls do you know who get this much calcium?

There are a few dietary habits that might make you lose calcium or not absorb it. A serious culprit that robs your body of calcium is carbonated sodas, either diet or regular. How many do you drink a day? Drinking two or more carbonated sodas containing phosphates a day inhibits calcium absorption. The phosphates in sodas bind to calcium in the intestine so that it cannot be absorbed by the body. Check the sodas you drink to see if they contain phosphates by checking the label for phosphoric acid. If you take in additional calcium through foods or supplements, you can offset the effect that a diet high in phosphates has on calcium balance. If you drink more than

Table 6.2

Calcium Contents of Common Foods

Food	Amount	Calcium (mg)
Whole milk	1 cup	291
Low-fat milk	1 cup	300
Skim milk	1 cup	302
Buttermilk	1 cup	285
American cheese	1 ounce	174
Cheddar cheese	1 ounce	204
Cottage cheese, large curd	1 cup	135
Cottage cheese, lowfat	1 cup	155
Mozzarella, part skim	1 ounce	207
Swiss cheese	1 ounce	272
Plain lowfat yogurt	8 ounces	415
Plain nonfat yogurt	8 ounces	452
Fruited lowfat yogurt	8 ounces	345
Vanilla ice milk or ice cream	1 cup	176
Sherbet	1 cup	103
Chicken breast	3$\frac{1}{2}$ ounces	15
Turkey, light meat	3$\frac{1}{2}$ ounces	20

Egg	1 large	25
Roast beef, eye round	3 ounces	4
Ground beef	3 ounces	9
Pork chop	3 ounces	4
Lamb, leg	3 ounces	7
Flounder	3 ounces	13
Red salmon	3 ounces	36
Pink salmon, with bones	3 ounces	167
Rainbow trout	3 ounces	73
Tuna, solid white	3 ounces	17
Lobster	3 ounces	52
Shrimp	3 ounces	33
Tofu	4 ounces	150
Almonds, whole	1 ounce	75
Brocolli	1/2 cup	47
Collard greens	1/2 cup	179
Kale	1/2 cup	90
Snap beans	1/2 cup	31

Nutrient data from J. Pennington, 1992, *Bowes and Church's Food Values of Portions Commonly Used,* 16th ed. (Philadelphia: Lippicott.) Reprinted, by permission, from N. Clark, 1997.

two cans a day of phosphate containing sodas, you need about 100 mg of additional calcium for each soda.

Very high protein intake can cause calcium to be excreted into the urine. Animal protein such as that found in beef, chicken, and fish appears to cause more calcium loss in the urine than the vegetable protein found in soy products. Exactly how much protein intake affects your calcium balance is not completely known. However, if more than 30 percent of your diet consists of protein, you may need to add extra calcium to stay in balance.

Try to determine how much calcium you need, and then decide how you will get that amount into your diet. Use table 6.2 and the calcium quiz below to determine your current calcium intake. Check table 6.1 (page 164), which lists your daily needs depending on your age and menstrual status. Getting this amount of calcium will not build bone, but it will supply your body with enough calcium to stay in balance.

◇Do You Get Enough Calcium?

Follow the steps to see if you eat and drink enough of these foods for strong bones.

Step 1: Take a minute to remember everything you ate yesterday at breakfast, lunch, dinner, and snacks.

Step 2: As you look at the list of high-calcium foods, write on the line next to each food how many servings you had yesterday. Make sure these are foods you *usually* eat. Remember that many things you eat contain a combination of foods. For example, a burrito may have tortillas, beans, and cheese. Be sure to include serving of combination foods. Put your number in the box at the bottom of the high-calcium food chart.

___ 1 cup nonfat, lowfat, or whole milk or buttermilk

___ 1 cup lowfat chocolate milk or hot chocolate

___ 1 cup nonfat or lowfat yogurt

___ 1½ ounce (about 1½ inch cube) lowfat or regular cheese

___ 1 cup milkshake

___ 1 cup pudding, custard, or flan

___ 6 sardines with bones

Number of high-calcium servings _____

Step 3: Look at the list of medium calcium foods. Write on the line next to each food how many servings you had yesterday.

Make sure these are foods that you *usually* eat. Remember that calcium is also added to foods that don't contain it naturally— such as orange juice, cereal, or bread. Be sure to read the label to include those foods. Put your number on the line at the bottom of the medium-calcium food chart.

__ 1/2 cup nonfat or lowfat cottage cheese

__ 1/2 cup cream soup

__ 1/2 cup ice milk, frozen yogurt, or ice cream

__ 1 cup dried beans or peas

__ 1 cup refried beans

__ 2 ounces canned fish, with bones (salmon, mackerel)

__ 1/2 cup tofu processed with calcium

__ 1/4 cup almonds

__ 1/2 cup bok choy or turnip greens

__ 1 cup broccoli, kale, or mustard greens

__ 5 figs

__ 2 corn tortillas

__ 1 tablespoon black strap molasses

__ 2 tablespoons nonfat cream cheese

Number of medium-calcium servings _____

Three medium-calcium servings equal one high-calcium serving. So if your medium-calcium servings equal

4, count as 1⅓ high-calcium serving;

3, count as 1 high-calcium serving;

2, count as 2/3 high-calcium serving; or

1, count as 1/3 high-calcium serving.

Now, write the number of medium-calcium servings as converted to high-calcium servings here _____

Step 4: Add the two values (from steps 2 and 3) here to find your total calcium servings _____

Step 5: Compare your total to the calcium servings you need.

The average American woman gets only about 400 to 600 mg of calcium a day. This means that most women are in calcium deficiency. The only way their bodies are maintaining calcium levels in their bloodstreams is by removing calcium from the bones.

How Can I Get Enough Calcium?

Now that you are convinced of the importance of getting enough calcium, how can you do this simply and effectively? You can incorporate dairy products, calcium-fortified foods, canned fish with bones, and some vegetables into your diet (see table 6.2). This is the best way to meet your calcium needs. Your body also needs vitamin D, which helps it absorb calcium and build bone. Vitamin D is taken in food or in supplements in the inactive form. It then requires you to be exposed to 15 minutes of sunlight each day to convert it into the active form.

A rule of thumb is that an average serving, about one cup of a dairy product, gives you 300 mg of calcium. Thus, just one serving of any dairy product with each of three meals almost meets your calcium needs. If you include some green vegetables in your diet, you will have no problem reaching your daily need for calcium. A nighttime snack that is calcium rich will provide the added boost for someone who needs more calcium. Some examples of calcium-rich snacks (300 mg each) are an 8-ounce glass of milk, a cup of yogurt or ice cream, or 1 ounce of cheese (approximately a 1 × 1 × 1-inch cube of cheese). If you can't tolerate or don't like dairy products, soy milk and fortified orange juice have the same amount of calcium as regular milk. Some power and energy bars are also fortified with calcium. If none of those foods sound appetizing, how about adding calcium or soy powder to a smoothie, adding tofu as a cheese substitute to pizza, making trail mix with calcium-rich almonds, or snacking on chocolate pudding or tapioca? Also, don't overlook veggies. Vegetables such as broccoli, kale, spinach, and Swiss chard contain calcium. However, the level of calcium in these foods is much lower than it is in dairy and soy products.

Some people do not like or cannot digest dairy products or choose to avoid them if they are vegan. Approximately 10 percent of the population has difficulty digesting the sugar naturally found in milk, known as lactose. Lactose intolerance can be an embarrassing condition. If you have this condition, you are likely to have uncomfortable bloating in the abdomen, gas, and diarrhea after eating milk products. The condition is diagnosed by a history of problems digesting milk or a specialized test done on your breath after drinking milk. You can still enjoy the health benefits of dairy products by choosing foods with the lactose removed. Lactose-free milk has all the calcium and nutritional value of regular milk and is available in most grocery stores. (It might taste slightly different.) You can also choose to take a tablet called Lactaid, which helps you digest lactose, whenever you choose to eat dairy products. Discuss this condition with your health care provider if you think you have it. And look for strategies to ensure your daily calcium intake in spite of it.

If you are a strict vegetarian, there are many appetizing options for you, beginning with the calcium-fortified juices and soy, rice, or even almond milk. Soy milk can be used to make smoothies or Popsicles and it can be added to creamed soups and mashed potatoes. Many vegetarians have found great recipes for tofu, a soy product that is very rich in calcium and can be used as a meat or cheese substitute. Vegetables that contain both calcium and oxalic acid may not be the best choice, because oxalic acid impairs the absorption of calcium. Swiss chard and spinach contain oxalic acid, but broccoli, kale, mustard greens, and bok choy are high-calcium veggies without the oxalic acid chaser.

If you find it difficult to meet your calcium needs, consider taking a calcium supplement. There are dozens of types, and all are available without a prescription. With all those choices, how do you decide which one is for you?

Not all calcium pills are created equal. Calcium has to be added to another element to get it into tablet form. Thus, you will see tablets labeled as calcium carbonate, calcium citrate, calcium gluconate, and calcium phosphate, to name a few. Only part of each tablet is calcium. For example, 40 percent of a calcium carbonate tablet is calcium, but calcium makes up only 21 percent of a calcium citrate tablet and just 9 percent of calcium gluconate tablet. We recommend taking calcium in a form that dissolves easily in your stomach and has a high amount of calcium in each pill. Calcium carbonate or calcium citrate supplements fit this description.

How can you tell how much calcium is in a tablet? Check the label for the amount of elemental calcium or the amount of calcium by weight. Table 6.3 shows the calcium content of various supplements. If the label says a tablet provides 1,000 mg of calcium carbonate, that tablet actually contains only 400 mg of calcium, because it is only 40 percent calcium. If the label of a supplement says it contains 400 mg of calcium, then it should contain 400 mg of calcium no matter the form it's in. When in doubt, ask the pharmacist or your health care provider.

Another thing to look for in a calcium supplement is whether or not it contains other minerals or substances that might be harmful. Recent reviews of calcium derived from bone meal (from animals), dolomite, and oyster shells has found that these sources of calcium might contain metal and mineral contaminants such as arsenic, lead,

Table 6.3

Percentage of Calcium Available in Various Supplements

Calcium source	Percent calcium by weight
Calcium carbonate	40%
Dicalcium phosphate	31%
Calcium citrate	21%
Calcium lactate	13%
Calcium gluconate	9%

Source: Tufts University Newsletter, April 1985

mercury, and cadmium. Even supplements that state they are "all natural" may contain these possibly harmful contaminants. The nonprofit Natural Resources Defense Council recently reported that many calcium supplements contained levels of lead that exceeded the levels considered safe in California (intakes of 0.5 micrograms a day). Federal levels for safe lead intake are set much higher, at 7.5 mcg a day. Lead is of concern because it can accumulate in the body and lead to heart disease, memory problems, high blood pressure, and kidney disorders. Pregnant women may pass along lead to their fetuses. Only 3 out of 25 supplements tested were almost lead free. They are Tums 500, Posture-D High-Potency Calcium, and Children's Mylanta Antacid. Watch for new technologies that are on the horizon to produce contaminant-free calcium supplements in the near future.

A further concern about calcium supplements is that they may not dissolve in your intestines so that the calcium can be absorbed and used by your body. Believe it or not, a lot of compressed tablets do not dissolve well in the stomach's acid and may pass out of the body without being absorbed. To test how well your calcium pill dissolves, put it in a glass with one part vinegar and three parts water, which mimics the acidic environment of your stomach. Leave it there for 20 minutes, then shake and see if it is dissolves the way it should in your stomach. It is best to take calcium supplements after a meal, when there is plenty of acid to help dissolve the tablet and speed absorption.

Another consideration is cost. Prices for calcium supplements vary from a few cents to more than a dollar per tablet. The most expensive is not necessarily the best. Low-cost options are generic or pharmacy-brand calcium carbonate or calcium citrate tablets. These are high in calcium and they are easily absorbed. Some of the Tums products, which are calcium carbonate, are also reasonably priced, free of contaminants, and easily absorbed. Flavored, chewable calcium supplements are available as well.

Calcium Supplements and Side Effects

Occasionally there are side effects from taking calcium supplements, such as gas, bloating, nausea, diarrhea, and constipation. You can avoid some of the side effects by slowly introducing calcium supplements; start with half a tablet and gradually build up to the amount you need. They are usually large pills, because calcium is a bulky mineral. If you have trouble swallowing large pills, choose a type that is chewable or powdered.

Calcium supplements may also cause kidney stones. If you take in more than 1,000 to 1,500 mg a day, the excess calcium is filtered out by your kidneys. If you don't drink enough water, it is possible that high amounts of calcium can form kidney stones. To be safe, drink plenty of water, at least an extra 8 ounces for each calcium tablet.

Roles of Other Essential Vitamins and Minerals

Add vitamin D, vitamin C, iron, zinc, magnesium, and other trace minerals to the list of nutrients essential to building bone. Calcium is the star of the show, but it needs a supporting cast to do its job well. As previously mentioned, to absorb calcium your body needs the active form of vitamin D. You can get vitamin D in fortified milk (cow or soy milk) or in a supplement that contains 400 to 800 I.U. (International Units) of vitamin D. A 15- to 20-minute walk in the sun will activate the vitamin D in your body. Trace minerals such as iron, zinc, and magnesium are just beginning to be studied for their bone-building effects. They are found in meat, oysters, crab, nuts, some dairy products, fortified cereals, and multimineral supplements. If you choose to take them in pill form, do not take a mineral supplement at the same time you take a tablet that contains calcium; the minerals in one tablet may block the absorption of the minerals in the other. You should take them at least two hours apart.

Research on postmenopausal women has shown that taking about 100 to 200 mg a day of vitamin C, in addition to calcium supplements, results in higher bone mass. You can add vitamin C to your diet with a serving of fruit, such as an orange, or a low-dose, up to 500 mg, vitamin C supplement. The specific way in which vitamin C works to build bone is not known.

Role of Hormones

Bone growth really takes off during puberty when the bones are exposed to the sex hormones, primarily testosterone in boys and estrogen in girls. These hormones (along with progesterone and androgens) are essential for the growth of a normal skeleton and for bone health throughout life. Men or women who lack or who have lower than normal levels of these hormones have been shown to quickly start losing bone mass. A wide variety of other hormones in the body (such as cortisol and thyroid hormone) have been evaluated in limited studies to see if they either benefit or harm bone.

Estrogen

Studies on young as well as older women convincingly show that without estrogen, between 1 and 5 percent of the total bone mineral density is lost per year. No wonder it is the most important factor throughout a woman's life in building strong bones. Estrogen works in three ways to help build bones and maintain dense bones.

1. It helps the body absorb calcium from the intestine. Given their typically low amounts of calcium intake, it seems women need all the help they can get.
2. Estrogen reduces calcium loss through the kidneys.
3. Most important, estrogen acts directly on the cells that remodel the bone, the osteoclasts and osteoblasts. When there is not enough estrogen, there is a loss of synchronization between the remodeling units of bone. Without estrogen's direct effect, osteoclasts take over, and bone resorption outpaces bone formation. The result is a loss of bone due to increased activity by the osteoclasts. When estrogen is present, it has a direct and immediate effect to slow down the osteoclasts' resorption of bone and results in less bone loss. There is also evidence that estrogen improves bone's response to exercise. Women who exercise and have normal levels of estrogen gain more bone than do women with low estrogen levels who exercise.

Thus, because of these three estrogen effects on calcium balance, women who are estrogen deficient need more calcium. Current recommendations are that estrogen-deficient women of all ages should get at least 1,500 mg a day. The estrogen effect is much greater than any other influence on bone mass. If exercise and calcium help bone by a factor of 2, then estrogen helps bone by a factor of 10.

Connecting Your Menstrual History to Your Bone Mass

Work done by Barbara Drinkwater, PhD, and others has shown that a woman's bone mass can be predicted based on her menstrual history. In one project, the subjects answered two questions about their menstrual histories and then had a bone mass measurement done. They were asked to describe their menstrual histories in one of three ways: amenorrhea for three months or more, irregular menstrual periods, or regular menstrual periods. They were then asked to describe what their menstrual cycles were like now, with the same three possibilities. Researchers could predict bone mass based on this information. The lowest bone mass is in women who both had a history of amenorrhea and were currently amenorrheic. The highest bone density was found in women who had always had regular periods.

Progesterone and Androgens

Progesterone is made during the two-week-long luteal phase of the menstrual cycle (see chapter 5, page 114). Several researchers have found that progesterone also has some bone-building action. In addition, the ovaries make small amounts of several different androgens, hormones found in larger amounts in males. Androgens such as testosterone clearly build bone in men and are the reason men have greater bone density than women. Further research is needed about the precise role these hormones play in women's bone health.

Cortisol

Excesses of certain hormones can cause bones to become osteoporotic. Cortisol, made by the adrenal gland, is a stress hormone that causes the rapid breakdown of bone without a compensatory increase in bone rebuilding. Any medical condition marked by high cortisol levels (Cushing's disease, overactivity of the adrenal gland) can also lead to osteoporosis. In addition, cortisol-like compounds are given as a medical treatment for certain illnesses (e.g., rheumatoid arthritis and asthma). Taking oral cortisone tablets for more than three months is associated with thinner bones. If you have been prescribed these medications in tablet, not inhaled form, and you have to take them on a regular basis, check with your physician about the possible impact on your bone growth.

Thyroid Hormone

Thyroid hormone is made by the thyroid gland, a butterfly-shaped gland in the neck. Excess thyroid hormone is known to be associated with bone loss. Higher-than-normal amounts of the hormone occur in a medical condition known as hyperthyroidism, or Grave's disease. Thyroid hormone may be prescribed for you as treatment for a medical condition such as hypothyroidism (low amounts of thyroid hormone). If you take the right amount, there is no harmful effect on your bones from thyroid hormone. However, if you take too much thyroid hormone, you will develop hyperthyroidism and lose bone mass. If you are taking thyroid hormone replacement, see your health care provider once a year to make sure that the dose is correct.

Role of Exercise

As you learned earlier in this chapter, bone that is exposed to enough calcium and estrogen responds and remodels according to the loads placed on it. The more the load, the denser the bone. Physical activity loads the skeleton in two ways:

1. by causing the muscles to pull on bones, and
2. by engaging the forces of gravity (if the activity is weight bearing).

For example, a gymnast lands in a tumbling routine with many times her body weight. Healthy bone responds by increasing its thickness and strength. If you do step aerobics, you get a great cardiovascular workout and a great bone-building workout, whereas if you take spinning classes, you only get a cardiac workout. A softball pitcher who uses her left arm for pitching generates a lot of muscular forces on the left side of her body. The bones on her left side get larger and thicker than those on her right side.

Exercise during childhood and puberty has a much greater bone-building benefit than exercise later in life. After puberty, exercise affects only the bones used and it must be in excess of your normal

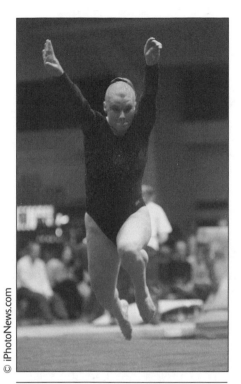

© iPhotoNews.com

Sports such as gymnastics can help build healthy bone if the athlete maintains an adequate calcium intake.

activity. Adults who stop exercising lose the bone mass they gained from physical activity. Gains made in puberty seem to stay with you for the rest of your life. Swimming and bicycling are wonderful exercise for the heart and lungs, but they do not have the bone-building effects of weight-bearing exercise. However, strength training, in addition to other weight-bearing exercise (e.g., running, aerobics, or any sport involving running, jumping, or walking), benefits the bones.

Exercise gives a mechanical stimulus to bones and increases bone formation by the osteoblasts. However, if you do not have enough building blocks for bone (such as calcium and Vitamin D) or enough estrogen, then your bones will not reap the benefits of physical activity. Bones facing a high mechanical load without the resources needed to build are at risk for breaking. Makes sense, doesn't it? If you don't build with the right materials, then when the earthquake comes, there is a greater chance for collapse.

The overall effects of exercise on bone were reviewed in the 1995 American College of Sports Medicine (ACSM) Position Stand.

ACSM Position Stand on Exercise and Osteoporosis

1. Weight-bearing activity is essential for the normal development and maintenance of a healthy skeleton. Increasing muscular strength may benefit nonweight-bearing bones such as the arms.

2. Sedentary women who become active may increase bone mass slightly, but the primary benefit of the increased activity may be in avoiding the rapid loss of bone that occurs with inactivity.

3. Exercise cannot be recommended as a substitute for hormone replacement therapy at the time of menopause or other times of estrogen deprivation.

4. For older women, exercise programs that increase strength, flexibility, and coordination may decrease the incidence of osteoporotic fractures by lessening the chance of falling.

BUILDING STRONG BONES THROUGHOUT LIFE

Since osteoporosis is preventable, what can you do throughout life to avoid this serious disease? There are different ways to maximize your bone mass, depending on your age. We have included bone-building guidelines for women of all ages.

Building Bone in Girls

The most important time to build strong bones that last the rest of your life is during your childhood and through puberty. The two most important things to do during this phase of life are to eat well and be active.

Many types of exercise are important in building the skeleton. We know that bone remodels according to the loads placed on it. Several clinical studies found that children who began physical training as early as age six had greater bone mass at the time of puberty than girls who did not. Studies on young gymnasts showed they had 20 percent more bone mass than their friends who were the same age but did not do gymnastics. Activities such as jumping and landing and tumbling build stronger bones than running. Here's a list of guidelines:

- ◆ Begin physical activity early in childhood. Choose activities you enjoy and that load the body in jumping and landing. These can include jump rope, tumbling, dance, gymnastics, basketball, volleyball, and jungle gym activities. Try to be active at least three times a week.
- ◆ Eat a well-balanced diet, following the guidelines of the food pyramid to ensure adequate protein, carbohydrate, and trace minerals.
- ◆ Ensure a daily intake of the bone builders—1,200 to 1,500 mg of calcium, 400 to 800 mg of vitamin D, 12 mg of zinc.
- ◆ Limit sodas containing phosphates. These can drain calcium out of the body.
- ◆ See a physician if puberty does not begin by age 14 or menstrual cycles do not begin by age 16.
- ◆ If you miss three or more menstrual cycles, see your physician.

Young Women and Bone Development

You only have about 70 percent of your genetically determined bone mass by the time you finish puberty (usually by age 18) and reach your adult height. The bone is long enough but not strong enough. From age 18 to 35, your bone is still growing and undergoing changes that will make it more dense and more able to withstand the demands of an active lifestyle. This is called skeletal consolidation. During this time, you continue to build an additional 30 percent of bone mass. What happens to your bones from puberty into your 30s is very important to your future. If you do not gain enough bone density, then you will be perilously close to the threshold for fractures for the rest of your life.

As you've learned, three things are critically important to build that skeleton: nutrition, exercise, and normal hormones. Of the three, having sufficient levels of female hormones to help build the skeleton is the most important by a factor of 10 times. Making sure you continue to have your periods is the single most important thing you can do to help maintain your bone mass!

Leah had done all the right things for her bones during her childhood. She had a mom who made her drink milk and eat yogurt and wouldn't allow many sodas. She did a lot of physical activity with her family and two older brothers. Bicycling, running, hopscotch, and kickball games were her favorites. When she was 8, she joined a gymnastics club after seeing the summer Olympics, and she declared that she wanted to be an Olympic gymnast. She stopped gymnastics when she discovered a love of running at age 10. She began running 10 km races with her brothers when she was 11, and she went to a summer running camp when she was 13.

Leah started having periods at age 15. Her mother remembered that her own periods seemed to have started late, at age 14½, but not having other daughters, she did not have anything to compare Leah's development to. When Leah was 17 and a high school senior trying to make it to the state meet, her coach encouraged her to lose weight. She started dieting and living on Diet Cokes and frozen yogurt. Her mother could not get her to eat with the rest of the family. She came home from track practice "too tired to eat anything heavy."

(continued)

When Leah went to college, and continued to diet, she stopped menstruating but did not tell anyone. She continued strict dieting along with one of her teammates and started throwing up after she ate anything "forbidden." Her freshman year, she had lost 10 pounds by the time she went home for winter break. Her mother was alarmed at her weight loss, but Leah reassured her that she was just getting in good shape. She worked out even harder over the winter break, running as much as 10 miles a day and doing speed work on a local track. She did not have energy for parties or for seeing high school friends.

Leah began having what she thought were shinsplints. She iced her legs every day and took pain killers. She tried new shoes with more cushioning. She thought she was too fat for the spring track uniforms, and she resisted all her mother's efforts to get her to eat her favorite foods. She made herself throw up a few times while she was home, after eating dinner with her family. When she returned to school, her shinsplints got worse. The college doctor diagnosed her with two stress fractures in one leg. She was told not to run for six to eight weeks. She was very upset at not being allowed to run. She didn't know what she could do stay in shape.

Devastated, she came home for spring break and decided to continue to work out for hours on the stationary bicycle. Thinner than she had ever been, Leah was grilled with questions by her mother. Leah denied anything was wrong and insisted that having stress fractures was "the price to pay" for being a runner. She told her mother that her periods had stopped but explained that "all the girls stop when they train hard."

Leah had done things right to build strong bones throughout her childhood, but during puberty there were indications that things were going wrong. Her periods started late, and she began dieting. During the critical years of bone growth, from ages 12 to 16, she did not have enough calcium or female hormones to ensure the normal growth of her skeleton.

After entering college, she increased her running, and her bones did their best to rebuild to meet the increased load. However, her bones did not get the calcium and estrogen they needed. Something had to give and it did; she developed two stress fractures. In Leah's case, when her bones should have been gaining in structure and density, they were actually losing mineral. She went for a bone density test and found that her bones were only 80 percent of normal.

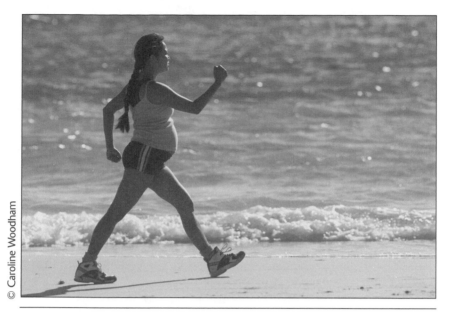

Pregnancy increases a woman's calcium needs to 1,500 mg a day.

Young women with amenorrhea and low estrogen levels lose as much as 1 to 5 percent of their total bone mass each year that they lack estrogen. The rate of bone loss is similar to the rate many women experience after menopause due to low estrogen levels, and it occurs even if women take adequate calcium. If you also have impaired nutrition, you may lose even more bone mass. Current research suggests that this bone loss is irreversible. Thus, if you have amenorrhea for two years, you may lose as much as 10 percent of your peak bone mass and may not be able to replace it. If you lose 10 percent of your bone mass, you increase your risk of stress fracture and osteoporosis.

Young adult women should know that pregnancy and breastfeeding also increase calcium needs. The calcium is needed to build the developing skeleton of the baby. Most prenatal vitamins contain some calcium, however its absorption may be blocked by the iron also found in these preparations. To get enough calcium for yourself and the growing baby, be certain you get 1,500 mg in addition to the prenatal vitamins. As discussed previously, food sources are best. With the increased calorie needs of pregnancy, you can make healthy choices by picking foods high in calcium (refer to table 6.2). If you do not get enough calcium from diet, consider taking a separate calcium supplement (see table 6.3).

The list on the following page summarizes guidelines to build strong bones for young adult women age 14 to 35.

◆ Participate in regular, weight-bearing activity to help maintain your bone mass. Up to age 30, exercise may help you gain bone mass and reach a higher peak bone bass. To be effective, exercise should be done regularly (three to five times a week). High-impact activities such as aerobics, dancing, team sports involving jumping and landing, some martial arts, stair climbing, running, and gymnastics-style tumbling are excellent choices.

◆ Add strength training to build muscle mass. Strength training is best done at least twice a week. Emphasize the major muscle groups of the trunk and legs such as the abdominal muscles, the spinal muscles, and the thigh muscles.

◆ Ensure adequate calcium intake of 1,000 to 1,500 mg a day. If you have amenorrhea, or are pregnant or breastfeeding, you need 1,500 mg a day.

◆ Seek medical care if your periods stop for three months or more. Amenorrhea can impair bone mineralization.

◆ Seek care immediately if you develop the early signs of an eating disorder. Eating disorders can lead to osteoporosis due to the lack of nutrition for the growing skeleton and their association with amenorrhea. Irreversible, permanent, deforming fractures of the bone have occurred in women with eating disorders.

Bone Maintenance: Ages 35 to 50

Women between 35 and 50 years old have been referred to as "the forgotten women" because of the lack of research and information on their health. What do we know now? During this period of life, you may have begun to lose some trabecular bone mass. Some studies have found a 7 to 16 percent loss of bone mass between the ages of 35 and 50. Getting enough calcium and exercise are important to keep the slow bone loss to a minimum. Women who are physically active, at least one hour per week, have higher bone mass than women the same age who do not exercise. Most women enter menopause between the ages of 42 and 55 and begin to lose bone mass because of lowered estrogen during this time. If your periods become irregular, or if you develop signs of menopause, such as hot flashes and infrequent periods, see your doctor. Until menopause, follow these general guidelines for healthy bones:

◆ Engage in regular, weight-bearing exercise; this can increase or maintain your bone mass. Aim for 30 minutes of exercise three to five times a week for at least four to six months to ensure some effect on bone.

◆ Add strength training to your exercise routine to help build bone mass and to increase strength. Two sessions a week, with emphasis on the large muscles of the trunk and legs, is best for bone stimulus. Focus on the muscles of the abdomen, back, and thighs.

◆ Seek medical care if your periods stop for three or more months.

◆ Ensure adequate calcium intake of 1,000 mg a day (1,500 mg a day if you have irregular menstrual cycles or are pregnant or breastfeeding).

Bone Protection During and After Menopause

It is well known that bone loss occurs after menopause. When a woman's periods stop, her ovaries no longer produce estrogen, progesterone, or the androgens. With the absence of the hormones come symptoms like hot flashes for some women, increased rates of coronary heart disease for most, and loss of bone mass for all.

Women lose one to five percent of their bone mass each year after menopause. A woman often does not know it is happening until her bones are thin enough that they break with a minor injury. If at any time in her life a woman reaches only 70 percent of her peak bone mass, she is likely to have a serious fracture with minor trauma. One factor that determines how quickly she gets to this fracture threshold is the peak bone mass she achieved earlier in life. If she only attained 80 percent of her predicted maximum, as is the case with Leah, she will be at fracture threshold (70 percent) within about two to three years after menopause.

However, women can take action after menopause to delay bone loss. Hormone replacement therapy is the single most important thing a menopausal woman can do to prevent bone loss. The following list provides additional guidelines.

◆ Engage in regular, weight-bearing exercise to slow bone loss. Exercise above and beyond your daily activities provides the maximum benefit. Try to perform 20 to 30 minutes of physical activity three to five times a week. Walking, jogging, dancing, aerobics, and stair climbing are among the best bone builders.

◆ Add strength training for the muscles of the arms, legs, and trunk. These exercises can be done two to four times a week with machines or home weights.

◆ See your health care provider to assess your risks for osteoporosis and other medical conditions. Decide what treatment is indicated based on this individualized assessment.

◆ Ensure that you get 1,500 mg of calcium each day if you are not taking estrogen replacement and 400 to 800 international units of vitamin D. If you are taking estrogen replacement, you need 1,000 mg of calcium a day.

DIAGNOSING AND HEALING A STRESS FRACTURE

The symptoms of a stress fracture are subtle. They start as a dull, aching pain that gets worse as activity continues. If you ice the area, rest, and take a few days off from weight-bearing exercise, the pain may go away. However, as soon as you resume activity, the pain returns. It may be particularly painful if you put all your weight on the afflicted bone. A bump may develop over the bone, and it may be very painful if you receive ultrasound treatments in physical therapy.

Because stress fractures are microscopic fractures, they do not show up on regular X-ray films immediately. They may be seen on X-rays two to eight weeks after the pain begins. What you see then is not the fracture, but rather the body's effort to repair the fracture with new bone. Due to the limitations of X-rays in early diagnosis of stress fractures, you may be referred for another type of test called a bone scan. A bone scan is not an X-ray, a bone density test (also known as a DXA; see page 190), or an MRI. It measures the activity of bone remodeling in the body. A bone scan will show a stress fracture within the first few days of pain. It involves injecting a small amount of a radioactive substance called technetium into the bloodstream. Technetium concentrates in any area of rapid bone turnover, such as a stress fracture. An MRI can also be used to diagnose stress fractures. Both tests must be ordered by a physician and read by a radiologist, a doctor who specializes in reading all types of imaging tests. These tests are expensive, and insurance may or may not cover them.

Stress fractures can be complex and chronic, particularly if you do not deal with them promptly and give them the time they need to heal. Furthermore, they can point to the more serious underlying condition of osteoporosis. A research study of college athletes found that at least one-third of the athletes with stress fractures lost an entire season due to the fracture and approximately half of them never returned to their prior level of competition.

If you have a stress fracture, make sure your physician checks for risk factors, using a questionnaire similar to the one on page 156, so your risk factors can be corrected if possible. If you have any of the components of the triad, let your doctor know so she can evaluate and treat these problems. Make sure you consult with a physician who has experience in sports medicine and stress fractures. She should take a careful history about your activity levels, running or playing surface, type of shoes, past and current menstrual patterns, and past and current eating habits. She should also ask questions that check your risk for stress fractures and low bone mass. She may suggest that you have your bone density measured (see pages 190 to 192).

Next, your physician should perform a physical examination that includes a check of your thyroid gland as well as a review of your gait (how you walk), your feet and lower legs, your lower body alignment and flexibility, and your shoes. If there are problems with your menstrual cycle, a full gynecological checkup will be done. If she finds significant abnormalities in your gait or foot examinations, she might refer you to a podiatrist or an orthopedic surgeon. Sometimes this team of doctors recommends custom-made inserts in shoes called orthotics, which correct the way your foot hits the ground and transmits loads up to your skeleton.

Other treatments for stress fractures may include physical therapy, gait retraining, nutritional review to ensure adequate calcium and mineral intake, and correction of any underlying risk factors. If you have amenorrhea as one of your risk factors, refer to the treatment section in chapter 5.

If you have a stress fracture, it is important to follow your physician's advice for treatment and time needed to heal the fracture. Most stress fractures take at least four to eight weeks to heal. When you return to activity, you need to start back slowly. Reduce the volume, intensity, and frequency of workouts from what you were doing before the stress fracture, then gradually increase the amount and intensity of training so your bone can successfully remodel itself instead of fracturing again. It may take a considerable period of time to get to your previous level of fitness or competition. As you recover from the stress fracture, you will need to have more time off to rest and rebuild after a workout. You may be advised to take every second or third day off training to give the bone a chance to rebuild. This is called a cyclic training schedule. Be sure you correct all your underlying risk factors and see your physician frequently if you have questions about your recovery time, therapy, or training.

At the very least, you will need to rest and reduce your weight-bearing activities for four to eight weeks to allow healing. Depending on the location of the fracture, you may be at risk for a complete fracture. Three serious sites of fracture are the tarsal navicular bone of the midfoot area, the neck of the femur (thigh bone) near the hip, and the front part of the tibia—the major bone of the lower leg.

If you have a stress fracture in any of those sites, there is a chance the bone will not heal or will go on to a complete fracture if you continue to put weight on it. Therefore, you may need to use crutches or have a cast or walking boot. In certain cases, a bone stimulation machine may be used to help heal fractures. Check with your physician to see if this will help you.

> Because she had two stress fractures, **Leah's** doctor referred her to a local university hospital for a bone mineral density test (DXA). The results showed she had a low bone density, nearly two standard deviations below normal for her age. How had this happened? She had a lower bone mass than other runners on her team because of her amenorrhea and consequent low estrogen levels. Thinner bones are more susceptible to stress fractures from the high loads that exercise creates.

> **Alexandra** did not have a history of amenorrhea or very high levels of exercise. What caused her stress fracture? She was a person who did too much too soon. She quickly went from being nearly sedentary to walking and doing aerobics. She also did not use appropriate shoes to protect her bones from the impact of new activities. Her doctor also decided to run a few tests to find out if there were any other reasons she might have gotten a stress fracture.

DIAGNOSING OSTEOPOROSIS

You now have a good idea what some of the risk factors for developing osteoporosis or stress fractures are. They are usually grouped into factors you cannot control—unmodifiable factors—and factors over which you have some control—modifiable risk factors.

One of the unmodifiable risk factors is your genetically determined peak bone mass level. For instance, certain racial groups have lower bone mass than others. Women who are Caucasian or Asian tend to have lower bone mass than Hispanic and African American women. Another relatively unmodifiable risk factor is your lifetime exposure to sunlight. Women who live in locations with little sunlight have increased rates of osteoporosis, because the body needs exposure to the sun in order to convert vitamin D to the active form that helps transport calcium into bone.

It is most important to find out if you have any risk factors that you can change now to benefit you in the future. Check the risk factors listed in table 6.4. If you have any risk factors, take action to correct them, or see a doctor for more treatment advice. Many of these risk factors will be familiar to you from what you have already learned about the female athlete triad and osteoporosis.

How many risk factors do you have? Can you take action now to correct these, or should you see a physician for an evaluation? If you can correct the risk factors of low calcium intake, smoking, or excessive alcohol intake on your own, great! If you need more information, see a nutritionist or health care provider for some guidance. Carefully review the guidelines on calcium intake (pages 164 to 168) to ensure that you are getting adequate calcium intake every day. If you are not, consider taking supplements.

Even with a careful history, a risk factor assessment, and a complete nutritional and physical examination, you still cannot be certain whether or not you have low bone mass. A bone density measurement test is the only way to be certain. This is best done in conjunction with seeing a physician who is experienced in the evaluation of women with low bone density. If you need to see a health care provider for concerns about osteoporosis, whom should you see? Your primary health care provider may be able to order and interpret osteoporosis tests. Most likely your physician will be familiar with this area if she is trained in internal medicine, pediatrics, adolescent medicine, family medicine, sports medicine, obstetrics and gynecology, or endocrinology. However, the treatment of young women with osteoporosis is a new field in medicine. Ask your physician if she has seen or managed a case of a young woman with osteoporosis. If not, ask for a referral to someone in your community who has. Many communities also have centers that specialize in osteoporosis or women's health. Doctors working in these specialized centers are likely to have the necessary expertise.

As with diagnosing a stress fracture, when you see the doctor, expect to give a history of your risk factors for osteoporosis. A physical examination should focus on screening for medical conditions that might result in osteoporosis. Your thyroid gland (located at the base of the front of the neck, above the top of the breastbone), will be examined. You

Table 6.4

Risk Factors for Osteoporosis

Factors you can't change

- Family history of osteoporosis (peak bone mass is 60 to 80 percent genetically determined)

- Racial background (Caucasian or Asian races are more susceptible to lower bone densities)

- Thin, ectomorphic body build

- Lack of exposure to sunshine due to climate

- Medical illnesses: hyperthyroidism, rheumatoid arthritis, diabetes, depression, connective tissue laxity syndromes (Ehlers-Danlos or Marfan Syndrome), hyperparathyroidism, Cushing's syndrome (high levels of cortisol)

- Chronic use and need for oral corticosteroids, antiseizure drugs

Factors you can change	Action to take to reduce risk
Inadequate calcium intake	Increase dietary calcium or supplement
Sedentary life style	Increase exercise, add weight training
Smoking	Stop smoking
High alcohol intake	Keep alcohol to 3 ounces a day
Excessive intake of coffee	Drink fewer than 3 cups a day
Consumption of phosphate-containing sodas	Lower soda intake or add calcium (100 mg for each soda)
Eating disorder	Ensure calcium intake, get medical care
Amenorrhea for more than 3 months	Get a medical evaluation, consume 1,500 mg a day calcium
History of oligomenorrhea	Get a medical evaluation, consume 1,500 mg a day calcium
Late menarche	Get a medical evaluation, consume 1,500 mg a day calcium
Medications	Discuss alternatives with physician

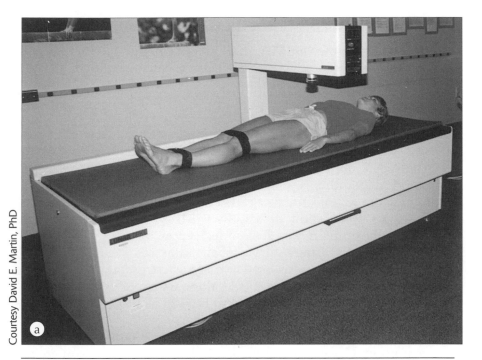

Courtesy David E. Martin, PhD

DXA tests are currently the safest and most reliable method of determining bone mineral density.

might have your height recorded and the looseness of your skin and joints tested as the doctor screens you for a condition of connective tissue laxity associated with osteoporosis. You will also be checked for any bone pain and for curvature of the spine (called scoliosis or kyphosis).

Your doctor will order blood tests to make sure that you do not have a medical problem that is causing osteoporosis. These include a test for thyroid hormone and for calcium and vitamin D levels in the bloodstream. Other tests may check the levels of hormones such as cortisol and parathyroid hormone, and kidney function. If you have amenorrhea, testing for this condition can be done at the same time (see chapter 5 for tests for amenorrhea).

The final diagnosis of osteoporosis is made by measuring your bone mineral density. There are several safe, reliable, and relatively inexpensive ways of measuring your bone mass and comparing it to what it should be.

Dual Energy Absorptiometry (DXA)

Currently, a test known as DXA, short for dual energy absorptiometry, is the safest and most reliable method for measuring your bone mass. This test is done by a machine that sends two low-energy X-ray beams through your bones while you lie under the machine on a special table. Usually, only the bone densities of the lower lumbar spine and the hip are measured. A computer compares your measured bone density to known standard bone densities of women your age. To have the test done, you just lie on a table that might be a bit hard and cold for 5 to 20 minutes while the X-ray is being done. There is no pain, there are no injections or pills to take, and there is very minimal exposure to radiation. In fact, there is less radiation than we are exposed to by sunlight. You feel perfectly fine after having this test done. This is test is different from a bone scan (see page 184), which involves an injection and is used to diagnose stress fractures.

In most states, you can have a DXA done with a referral from your health care provider. The average cost is $125 to $200. The test may or may not be covered by insurance carriers.

The results from this test are presented in a graph showing the curve of normal bone density (figure 6.5). You can see if you are in

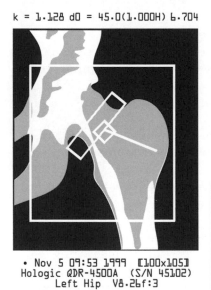

Region	BMD	T	Z
Neck	0.851	+0.02 100% (25.0)	+0.02 100%
Troch	0.681	0.22 97% (25.0)	0.22 97%
Inter	1.040	0.39 95% (35.0)	0.30 96%
TOTAL	0.911	0.25 97% (25.0)	0.25 97%
Ward's	0.784	+0.43 107% (25.0)	+0.43 107%

• Age and sex matched   T = peak BMD matched   Z = age matched

Figure 6.5 Sample report from a DXA test on a 23-year old woman. Her bone mineral density is slightly below the norms set for her age and sex.

the normal range or not. There is also written information about the actual measurement of the bone density (listed in grams per square centimeter) and two scores of your bone density. The first score, called the T score, compares your bone mineral density to that of a woman at age 30—presumably, the peak bone density. The second score is called the z score, and it compares your bone density to that of other women your age. If either your z or your T score is plus or minus one standard deviation (1 STD), then it is in the normal range. Statistically, 68 percent of people will be within 1 STD, either above or below the normal mark. Your doctor will help you interpret the results of this test for your particular situation.

If your values are more than 1 STD below normal, then you are at some risk for osteoporosis. If you are 2.5 or more STD below normal for your age on the z score, then you have osteoporosis and are at high risk of fracture. If you have a result that indicates you have lost bone mineral density, be sure and get a careful medical evaluation and assessment of your risk. Armed with the knowledge of your bone density, you will have control and power over your future risk of osteoporosis and fracture.

Knowledge can indeed be power in this situation. The bone mineral density measurement represents just one point in time. If you can make some changes in the factors that resulted in your loss of bone mineral density, you can see it increase or stabilize and you can avoid further loss. If your bone density is low, there are many good treatment options. Because the treatment is specific for each person, we advise that you discuss all your questions with and get answers from your referring physician.

There are some newly developed machines that test bone density using the same principles as the larger DXA machines. However, instead of measuring the spine or the hip, they measure the heel, wrist, or hand. The procedure is called single-energy photon absorptiometry (SPA) or dual-energy photon absorptiometry (DPA). These methods are inexpensive and may not require a physician referral. You may have been offered one of these tests at a health fair, a fitness club, or even at a pharmacy. The measurement from these machines is not as accurate as the DXA measurements taken at the hip and spine. They have been approved by the FDA for screening for osteoporosis, but not for diagnosis. If you are tested on any of these small screening machines and have a concern about the results, you should be referred to a specialist in osteoporosis.

X-Ray

There are techniques other than DXA to measure bone mineral density. A regular X-ray has been used. X-rays, such as those taken of your chest or bones, do not detect osteoporosis until a very late stage. You must have lost about 30 percent of your bone mass before changes appear on X-rays. This is dangerously low bone density, right at the fracture threshold. See a specialist if you have been told that a regular X-ray suggests osteoporosis.

Quantitated Computer Tomography

Quantitated computer tomography (known as QCT) is a fairly reliable test for bone density, particularly in young women. It uses higher energy X-ray beams to measure the bone density. It costs more than DXA and exposes you to more radiation.

TREATING LOW BONE DENSITY

There is no one specific treatment for low bone mass. There are several different approaches to improving bone mass depending on your age, the type of osteoporosis you have, and your underlying risk factors. If you have low bone mass, it is important to determine the cause so that specific treatment can be advised. Correcting the cause will give you the best chance of increasing or stabilizing your bone density.

In addition to getting enough calcium and other minerals (see pages 170 through 174), there are several treatment options under study for young women with low bone densities. The best option if you have amenorrhea is to make the lifestyle changes necessary to resume normal menstruation. If you cannot resume menstruation on your own, hormone replacement therapy may be an effective option. You can take estrogen and progesterone either in a single birth control pill or as two separate pills (see treatment of amenorrhea in chapter 5, pages 148 through 149). Current research suggests that birth control pills with more than 25 mcg of estrogen contain an adequate dose to stop bone loss. The postmenopausal hormone replacement therapies (e.g., Premarin and Provera) do not contain high enough levels of hormones to preserve bone in young women and also do not provide contraception. Some preliminary research suggests that if you use birth control pills for more than one year you may gain back some of the lost bone. However, once you stop taking these hormones, you will again be losing bone if you do not resume menstruation.

Fosamax (alendronate), a bone-building medicine, has been approved by the FDA for postmenopausal women, but it has not been approved for women of childbearing ages because it has a long half-life in the body, as long as 18 years. Another treatment that has been

Leah's primary care doctor referred her to an osteoporosis specialist to help decide what treatment she needed. Because she had two stress fractures, low bone mass, and the triad disorders, her doctor formed a multidisciplinary team to help with her treatment. She was put on birth control pills to increase her levels of estrogen and progesterone, and she was given a calcium supplement. A psychologist helped her develop coping skills to deal with her injuries, her dieting behavior, and her self-esteem. Leah met with the psychologist weekly and kept a journal about her struggle to get healthy.

Leah could not run because of the stress fracture and was completely bored with riding the stationary bike. She decided to concentrate on her schoolwork. She wrote a paper for one of her classes about osteoporosis and started telling her friends and teammates about the importance of calcium. She made smoothies with soy milk powder and carried around calcium-fortified energy bars. She worked with the psychologist on building a better body image and not worrying so much about her weight.

Leah was frustrated by the slow progress. Her doctor told her that because of her low bone density and amenorrhea, it might take quite a while to heal. For someone who was used to being fast and doing things quickly, the slow pace of her healing was hard to take. The psychologist helped her put her energy into other activities and learn patience. It took twelve weeks of not running to heal the two stress fractures.

Leah decided not to run on the team her sophomore year in college, and she worked harder in school. Her grades showed it. She gained back 10 pounds of the 15 she had lost and had a repeat bone density test done 18 months after her first one. She had gained 2 percent of bone mass so that she was now at 82 percent of the predicted bone mass for her age. Because she had actually gained back some bone mass, she stopped her birth control pills and her menstrual periods resumed naturally. Leah still missed not running track and hoped to return to it in her junior year. But she found a lot of other things about college that she liked, and she thought about heading for a career in health education or nutrition.

used in young women is calcitonin. It is derived from a hormone that is known to build bone and is given by injection or nasal spray. To date, calcitonin has not been shown effective in significantly increasing bone mass in premenopausal women. It may help decrease bone loss and preserve bone. Discuss all these options with your physician.

The length of treatment depends on what is causing your low bone mass and the type of therapy your health care provider recommends. Most of the treatment plans involve a treatment period and then a reassessment period to see if it is working. If you have had low bone mineral density measurements done, your physician may request a repeat test to see if your density has stabilized or increased. The range of error of the DXA is between 2 and 5 percent. The changes in your bone mineral density with treatment range between 1 and 5 percent a year. So it may take 12 to 18 months to see if any significant changes are occurring.

Good luck! With the knowledge you have gained by reading this chapter, you are well on the way to preventing stress fractures and osteoporosis. Share the knowledge with others (see chapter 8), and you can help your friends and family members also prevent old bones in young women.

WHAT LEAH'S AND ALEXANDRA'S EXPERIENCES TEACH US

As a child, Leah had a high calcium intake, which helped her build strong bones. Getting 1,500 mg of calcium a day as a child helped her maximize bone development. She was also physically active as a child, doing activities like gymnastics that included a lot of jumping and landing. High-impact physical activity helped her build strong bones. Leah's menstrual cycle started late, at age 15. The late start delayed her exposure to female hormones and may have impaired maximum bone development. Alexandra rapidly increased her level of exercise without medical advice.

Reduce your intake of phosphate containing sodas.

As a teenager, Leah began dieting and drinking phosphate-containing sodas. Her calcium intake dropped. Bone mineralization and density can be decreased if a girl does not get 1,200 mg of calcium a day during adolescence.

Action to take: Sodas containing phosphate may pull calcium out of the body, so extra calcium is needed, through diet or supplements, to replace what is lost. Recommendations are an additional 100 mg of calcium for every 8-ounce soda.

Make sure you have regular menstrual cycles.

At age 17, Leah stopped having menstrual periods. She did not go for a medical evaluation, which is recommended whenever a woman misses three menstrual cycles in a row, and did not increase her calcium intake.

Action to take: If you stop having your periods, see your doctor to determine the cause. You should also increase your calcium intake to 1,500 mg, which is the recommended intake for women who have amenorrhea and lack estrogen.

Stress fractures can be the first sign of osteoporosis.

Leah developed stress fractures when she increased her training. Her bones were already weaker than they should have been because of the effects of dieting and amenorrhea. When Leah was diagnosed with stress fractures, she had a thorough medical evaluation that included bone density measurements, training and nutritional assessments, and a gynecological evaluation.

Action to take: If you have a stress fracture, make sure your physician evaluates your bone health. This may include answering questions about your menstrual cycle, nutrition, and training. If indicated, a test to measure your bone density can be done. Do all you can to ensure bone health by getting adequate calcium, having regular menstrual cycles, avoiding disordered eating practices, and adding strength training.

Stress fractures can be a sign of overtraining.

Leah developed stress fractures when she increased her training. She increased her training by adding both distance and speed work at the same time, and this was too much too soon. Her bones were already weaker than they should have been because of the effects of dieting and amenorrhea.

Action to take: Never increase both the distance and intensity of your work outs at the same time. Look for gradual improvement over time and make sure you vary the intensity of your workouts. Avoid two intense workouts in a row. Don't forget you build muscle and strength when you are resting, not when you are exercising.

Missing your periods is not normal.

Leah thought that amenorrhea was normal and a sign that she was reaching peak fitness. This delayed her seeking treatment, and allowed her situation to get worse. In her case, the lack of menstrual periods was due to the energy drain of dieting and too much training, and it set her up for having stress fractures.

Action to take: In fact, amenorrhea is a sign that something is going seriously wrong in the body. A full medical evaluation is recommended.

If you have a stress fracture, learn how to train around it and keep a positive attitude.

When Leah was diagnosed with two stress fractures, she was devastated. However she did not give up or self-destruct. She began training on a bicycle to keep her cardiovascular system conditioned. With the help of the psychologist on her treatment team, she refocused her energy on schoolwork, she learned patience, and she improved her body image. Alexandra adjusted her exercise program and calcium intake when her stress fracture was diagnosed.

Action to take: Make sure you follow your doctor's recommendations to make sure you heal the fracture. Keep yourself fit with nonweight-bearing aerobic activity, such as swimming, pool running, rowing, or bike riding. Be honest about your feelings and seek counseling to help you with depression, anxiety or disordered eating.

Get treatment for the underlying causes of your stress fracture.

Leah started treatment for the underlying causes of her stress fractures—amenorrhea and disordered eating. By getting treatment early, Leah escaped the quicksand of a poor body image, self-destructive dieting, and disordered eating. While she was amenorrheic, she protected her bones by taking replacement hormones. She was able to correct some of the underlying dynamics that drove her to excessive dieting and weight loss. By the time her stress fractures had healed, she was a healthier person who was able to enjoy life and physical activity. Alexandra followed her doctor's advice to have some tests run to investigate possible reasons for her stress fracture.

Action to take: If you have a stress fracture, make sure you get evaluated and treated for any amenorrhea or disordered eating patterns. See chapter 7.

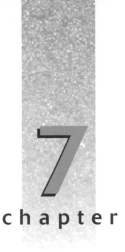

chapter

Getting Help:
Teamwork
for Success

If you recognize yourself or a friend in the stories of Leah, Jessica, Winnie, and Deborah, or in the experiences of the other women's presented in this book, don't hide, despair, or self-destruct. You can overcome an extreme drive for thinness and disordered eating, and the consequent amenorrhea and bone density losses that can occur with them. There are abundant resources to help. And where there is help, there is hope. Because these disorders are chronic, it may take time to get better. Be patient. These disorders are complex, so you may need help from several different experts. Going for help may not be easy. You must have the wisdom to recognize that you need help, the support to go, and the strength to get better, stronger, and healthy again.

Kathy was an excellent student in high school. She had many friends and was on the swim team. She went to college as a premed student on an academic scholarship. Her parents expected her to be a doctor or a lawyer. She had a younger brother and older sister, all of whom grew up competing against each other, particularly in swimming. When she started college in a town 400 miles away from home, she missed her friends and her sister. She hardly knew anyone in her premed classes. She decided to try out for the swim team and join a sorority.

She made the swim team as a walk-on. She found that many of her sorority sisters were different from her friends in high school. They all seemed very focused on meeting guys and were dieting and talking about losing weight all the time. By the time of the fall quarter midterms, Kathy had not been asked out on one date. She decided she needed a new look to fit into the college scene, and she started to diet. Her swimming teammates were also dieting to swim faster and to make the weight the coach expected of them at weigh-ins each Monday. Kathy found that if she had only Diet Cokes and frozen yogurt on Sunday, she could always make her weight for swim practice on Monday. She was not the best swimmer, but she was the best at losing weight.

At Monday night sorority meetings, when cookies were served, she had more willpower than most of her sorority sisters. She started weighing herself several times a day. Although lonely, she felt a sense of accomplishment and felt good about herself whenever she lost another pound. When she came home for the holiday break, her parents and high school friends were impressed at how lean she was. Her mother had always stressed being thin as a way of being accepted and attractive. She took Kathy shopping for new clothes, in a size smaller than she had ever fit in before. Kathy had more energy than ever.

In January, Kathy was delighted when she stopped having her menstrual periods and the monthly bloated feeling that went with them. The scale became her friend as she continued to lose about a half-pound a week. Sometimes she lost more if she was really good and cut out all fat in what she ate. She still found it hard to meet guys, and she didn't like going to fraternity parties where everyone seemed to drink a lot. Her premed classes were difficult, and her grades weren't as good as they had been in high school, so she stayed away from most social activities to study more. She wasn't dating and found she did not have much in common with her sorority sisters, who were planning formal dances and weekend getaways with fraternities. In April, she stopped eating in the sorority and ate only in her room so that she wasn't tempted to eat too much. She mainly ate yogurt and cereal while she studied. She counted how many Cheerios she ate and kept it strictly at 100 for breakfast.

Studying for finals at the end of the year, she gave in and ate two slices of a pizza that was delivered to a study group. After eating it, she felt gross, disgusted, and nervous. She left the study group and went upstairs to her room to weigh herself. She had gained two pounds from eating that pizza! She resolved to be more strict the next week and not eat at all for a day. Making that resolution, she felt better for awhile. She would never eat pizza again!

When she went home for the summer, her mother noticed that she had lost more weight and her new clothes seemed too big for her. She seemed irritable and prone to argue. She worked out at the club, swimming every day. High school friends called her, but she usually did not do things with them, unless it was to shop or go to a movie (where she brought her own fat-free popcorn to eat). Her older sister, Angie, was also home for the summer and noticed these changes. She told Kathy she was worried about her. Kathy said that there was nothing wrong and secretly thought her sister was jealous of how thin she was.

RECOGNIZING THAT YOU NEED HELP

Recognizing that you need help is the first, most important, and most difficult part of your journey to recovery. Why is recognizing that you need help the first step? To recover from any part of the female athlete triad, you must see that you have a problem. Be realistic enough to realize that you need the help of others to become healthy again. Be honest enough to see that you are doing something harmful to yourself. You might have mistakenly been told that the symptoms of the triad you've been experiencing are part of normal physical training. Learning that this is not true can motivate you to go for treatment.

On the other hand, you may be in denial, as are many women who suffer from the triad disorders. They are unwilling or unable to recognize that there is anything wrong. If this is your case, then to get help you first need to lift the veil of denial, secrecy, self-control, and shame that you may feel about your behaviors and body. To do this, you must connect to the part of yourself that is healthy. This is the part of you that was there before you developed disordered eating and knows disordered eating behavior is harmful. If you are embarrassed, in hiding, or in denial, the first step of recognition may take weeks, months, or years. It may take repeated efforts by your friends, family, and others to point out that what you are doing to yourself is not healthy and that you have a problem. However, you can stop disordered eating behaviors from controlling your life. Begin the battle to recover and regain your true self.

Recognizing that you need help is an important step because it means you have started to face reality. It is now possible for you to manage your eating disorder, amenorrhea, and low bone density instead of the other way around. Awareness of the problem is the most important predictor that you will get better. Your ability to go for help is the most important sign that you have the strength and courage to heal and save yourself from the serious consequences of the triad. You can build a positive self-image and a life filled with happiness.

It can be incredibly difficult to admit that you have a problem and that you can't conquer it alone. Most women who develop triad disorders are accustomed to being successful. You have probably tried to stop purging or obsessing about every calorie you eat. Every month you might have hoped your period would come back or taken a lot of calcium to try to ward off osteoporosis. Because you've been unable to correct the conditions of the triad by yourself, you may feel like a failure. But you aren't. Recovery takes help from others.

Perhaps your friends and families responded positively when you first started losing weight. Perhaps your running times improved, or you were able to jump higher or move faster on the playing field for a while. At first, your dieting or new eating practices were seen falsely as an accomplishment. You might have been encouraged to become thinner, and you might have thought that losing your period was a sign that you were doing the right things. For some of you, these behaviors are difficult to confront, because they have become a part of your identity or a way of coping with pressures and problems. Admitting that you need help can also be difficult because it may mean dropping rigid self-control and

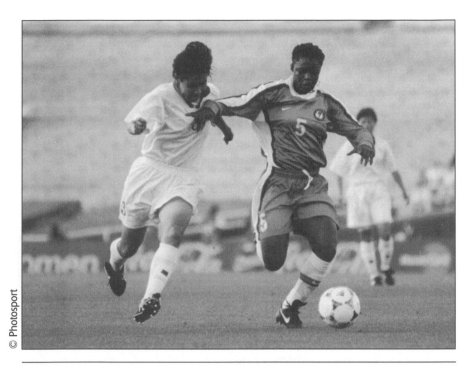

Strong, physically fit women are now role models for women, replacing the thin fashion models.

developing a different way of living and of looking at yourself and your body. It may be frightening to think about eating differently, gaining some weight, or getting a dreaded menstrual period.

Noticing the Signs

You now know some of the physical and psychological problems associated with the triad. If you have any of the following signs you need to seek treatment.

Physical Symptoms

- ◆ You have had amenorrhea for three or more months
- ◆ You have cardiac symptoms such as irregular pulse, skipped heartbeats, or very slow pulse
- ◆ You have passed out (fainted)
- ◆ You see blood when you vomit
- ◆ You use disordered eating practices on a regular basis
- ◆ You lose two or more pounds a week due to disordered eating

♦ You have lost more than 10 percent of the expected body weight range for your age and height

Psychological Symptoms

♦ You have considered taking your own life
♦ You feel depressed, hopeless, and anxious, or you cry often
♦ You have tried to stop bingeing and purging, but cannot
♦ You continue to exercise even when injured
♦ Your friends or family are worried about you and urge you to get help
♦ You are preoccupied by thoughts about food and weight control

When **Kathy** went home during the summer after her first year in college, she found it harder to lose weight. She had been so successful at this in school! She tried eating less and began running in place in her room, in addition to swimming. She went to summer school chemistry class four hours a day and worked in a bank part-time. Every other spare moment was taken up with her new plan to lose weight and get in shape. Kathy liked to weigh herself in order to reassure herself that she was getting thinner. Although she had lost 20 pounds in her first year in college, and at 5'6" had gone from 130 pounds to 110 pounds, she felt fat, especially in her hips and stomach. Her goal was to weigh 100 pounds or less. She did not like going out with friends, because they seemed to waste a lot of time and end up eating pizza or other meals that were "too heavy."

If she did not work out twice a day, she felt anxious and got mad at herself for not having enough discipline. Her parents, who at first had been impressed at her weight loss, were now concerned about her thinness and about how withdrawn she was from friends and family. Kathy resented the fact that they asked her constantly about her weight and forced her to eat with them at family dinners.

A few times during her swim workouts, she had to stop because it felt like her heart was beating so fast it would come out of her chest. She thought she was out of shape and re-solved to do more sprints. Her high school friends all talked about what a great time they'd had in college and how they couldn't wait to go back. Kathy couldn't wait to get back as well, but it was because she felt she was in prison at home and wanted to go back to school where she felt more in control.

Kathy's older sister, Angie, found Kathy really different and not as much fun to be around. Angie had taken a psychology class and was worried that Kathy had the signs of depression or anorexia. She told Kathy she was worried about her. Kathy laughed at her and saw her sister as being resentful of how thin and attractive Kathy was. Angie had gained 15 pounds her first year in college, and their mother had made Angie go on a diet. Kathy secretly ran in place in her room for 45 minutes each night. Sometimes she felt her heart racing, but she just stopped for a few minutes until her heart rate went back down.

Can't I Stop This Myself?

A common misunderstanding is that you can simply stop the disordered eating or compulsive exercising by deciding you will. Many times parents, friends, and even coaches of girls and women with eating disorders ask me, "She knows that it is harmful to her; why doesn't she just stop?" If you have tried to stop but cannot, you already know it is not easy. Eating disorders are complex behaviors that may be addictive. They may also be your only mechanism for dealing with stress.

When I talk to parents or friends about how hard it is to voluntarily stop eating disorders, I compare the disorders to fingernail chewing or cigarette smoking. Both are behaviors that embarrass people and that they would like to stop. But as anyone who has tried to stop chewing their fingernails or stop smoking knows, it is incredibly difficult. Once a behavior pattern is started, it is hard to change, particularly by just willing yourself to stop. Disordered eating is very difficult, if not impossible, to stop without professional help. It is a self-perpetuating behavior, one that has a life of its own irrespective of insight and the will to stop. Disordered eating often is a way of coping with underlying psychological problems.

Why Get Treatment?

Why go through all of the agony of recognizing that you need help? Because in the long run, it will be worth it. You will take the first steps toward saving your life, recovering your true self, improving your energy and body image, freeing up your time, and becoming interested in things other than food and exercise. You will be taking action to correct any medical problems, protect your bones from osteoporosis, save your heart from damage due to starvation or bulimia, preserve your tooth enamel, and guard your digestive system from the ravages of disordered eating. By getting treatment, you'll regain your menstrual periods and your sexual desire, and you may improve your chances of being able to have children. Your academic and work performance will improve. If you are anxious or depressed, you are likely to feel better. If you have had problems in relationships, they are likely to improve. Your athletic performance will improve, and you'll have the energy to train more effectively.

Kathy's sister, Angie, continued to worry about her. Kathy had always been a fun, outgoing person, and the smartest one in the family. Now she was angry, depressed, and irritable. And Angie knew that Kathy had stopped having her menstrual periods, because when she asked to borrow some tampons, Kathy told her, "I don't have any because I don't have my period any more." From what she had learned in her psychology classes, Angie thought Kathy might have anorexia. Kathy also had read about the female athlete triad in a women's sport magazine. Angie tried talking to Kathy, telling her she thought Kathy was too thin and might have anorexia. This attempt backfired, and Kathy angrily ran out of the room and slammed the door.

Angie contacted her psychology professor to get some more information about anorexia and the triad. He suggested a few books and gave her contact information for the American College of Sports Medicine for information about the triad and the local chapter of Anorexia Nervosa and Related Eating Disorders, Inc. He also gave her the names of two clinical psychologists and two medical doctors in her hometown who were experienced with these problems. Angie recognized one of the doctors as the physician for their high school swim team. The professor told Angie it was likely that Kathy's problems had taken a while to develop and that they would not change overnight. He encouraged Angie to be patient and to continue to be caring and concerned about her sister until Kathy was ready to open up and go for help. In the meantime, Angie read and learned more about the triad.

If the eating disorder is a symptom of another problem, you can help yourself acheive long-term health by dealing with that underlying problem. The earlier you get treatment, the more likely it is that you will have a good outcome and recover your health and happiness. You will also benefit from better athletic performance when you correct your energy deficiency. You will avoid some of the pitfalls of the female athlete triad (e.g., stress fracture), and you will have the energy to perform at your best.

Hannah is a 30-year-old high school teacher. Concerned, she came to see me about her friend Janice. She said, "I have taught with Janice for three years, and for the past year, she has had a lot of problems with her weight. Her parents live out of town, but she always talks about how her mom used to be a model and how hard it was to live up to her mother's expectations of her. Her weight bounces up and down and she is always talking about how fat she is, even though she looks fine to me. She works out erratically, sometimes exercising for two hours a day and then doing nothing for weeks. If we go out to eat with friends, she always excuses herself right after the meal to go to the bathroom, and we think she is vomiting. She gets down on herself a lot and isn't as much fun as she used to be. I talked to her a few times but she just brushed me off, and now she won't talk to me. I am really worried about her, and I want to do something to help."

HELPING A FRIEND

Hannah's and Angie's experiences with their friends and family members are very typical. Most women with the female athlete triad do not want others to know about their disorders and will resist caring efforts by friends or families to help them. They may act defensive and deny that anything is wrong. Even with all the education about the risks and the reasons for treatment, many women are unwilling to admit they have a problem, much less get treatment. Many women are afraid, ashamed, and unable to recognize how much the disorders have affected them and everything they do in their lives, including their training. The triad may seem so intertwined in their lives that it seems impossible to live without it. Maintaining an eating disorder to stay thin, or equating her thinness with her athletic successes may constitute a woman's identity, her way of coping with stress, or her notion of being in shape or attractive. Having amenorrhea may be a badge of honor that indicates she is training hard enough. Until the effects of the triad lose their usefulness for them or there is a serious frightening medical problem, many women are unlikely to get treatment.

What can you do if you are worried about a friend, family member, or teammate you think may have or be in the beginning stages of the female athlete triad? There is no one answer, but there are several possible approaches that you can take.

Educate Yourself

First, as Angie did, educate yourself. This doesn't mean writing a term paper; reading a few books, reading the articles recommended in this book's resources section, or contacting the local chapter of an eating disorder group are all good ways of getting information. Learning about these disorders can help you understand your friend or family member and her reluctance to get help. You can also speak with professionals who deal with the triad disorders (see p. 210 this chapter for more information on the type of professional to talk to).

Talk to Your Friend

When you are ready, willing, and able, speak directly to your friend or family member. Do not spread rumors or go around asking all her friends what they think. This is a way to lose the person's trust. How do you talk to her? There is no one right or wrong way. You will have to find what fits with your style and do it as honestly and naturally as possible. The approach we recommend is that of consistent, caring communication. Show you really care about the person and are willing to communicate about what concerns you. When you state your concerns, speak naturally and genuinely. Do not accuse, act judgmental, or make her feel guilty. Always talk to her in a private setting where you are sure you will not be overheard or interrupted. Choose a time when you won't be rushed. Your friend needs to know that she has privacy and confidentiality with you.

> After talking to **Hannah** about her friend Janice, I recommended that she read a few handouts I gave her about the triad and eating disorders and then arrange to get together with Janice at a time and place that would be comfortable for both of them. I told Hannah her best approach was to be herself and to speak honestly with Janice about her concerns.

Hannah told me specifically what worried her about Janice's behavior, and we jotted down a few ways that she could address these concerns to Janice using "I" statements. Hannah decided to start by letting Janice know how much she liked her, how much she admired her for her teaching skills and her sense of fair play, and how much fun she was to be with. Hannah would then tell her that she had noticed a change and wondered if Janice had been having any problems. Hannah also had referrals to give to Janice if she opened up. I told Hannah it was not her responsibility to diagnose or treat Janice, but to help her get to treatment.

When you speak to your friend or family member, do not analyze her or play amateur psychologist. You are her friend. You honestly care about her happiness and health. The easiest thing to do is to share your observations and concerns, emphasizing your positive feelings for her. The most direct and simplest way to do this is to use "I" statements in which you state what you have seen, been concerned about, or observed. "I" statements allow you to honestly state your worries without putting the other person on the defensive. You might say something like the following:

I am worried about you, because you seem so down all the time.

I'm really concerned that you are struggling with your weight, diet, or training, and I'm worried about you.

I know you have stopped having your menstrual period, and from what I know this is not normal. I hear it is a sign of a possible problem.

I know some people can get frustrated with dieting, and I am worried that is happening with you.

I just did some reading about eating disorders, and I am worried that you have one, because I heard you throwing up the other night.

I know you have a lot of pressure from your mom to be thin like she was. Can we talk about it?

By using "I" statements, you stick with what you really know and you speak from your heart. Try it; it works! And if it doesn't seem like the most natural way for you to speak, consider practicing it in front of a mirror or jotting down a few statements that you feel are honest and comfortable for you to use.

What might happen? Sometimes, the person is ready and will open up to you. Most likely, she will respond to your concerns with denial, no matter how caring your communication is. Don't take it personally. Remember that eating disorders are associated with a lot of denial, shame, and secrecy. Be prepared to hear denial, and restate your concern and caring for the person: I hear that you don't think you have a problem, and I just want you to know that I really care about you. That's why I brought this up.

> When **Hannah** decided to talk to Janice about her concerns, she chose a quiet, private place. They went for a walk in a nearby park that was a Japanese garden. Next to a Koi pond, they sat on a bench and talked about how beautiful the different-colored fish were. Hannah said, "I am concerned about all the changes you've been going through. How are you doing?" This was their second talk in the park, and Janice could see that Hannah really cared. She felt comfortable enough to open up to Hannah and agreed to go for a medical checkup.
>
> A week or two later, I saw that Hannah and Janice were on my clinic schedule. They came in together. Hannah said that Janice had some problems she wanted to discuss with me and that she had come along for moral support. Janice talked about her struggles with stress and the demands of teaching. She had trouble with eating and with her periods. Together, we worked out a plan of action. Two months later, Janice was doing much better, meeting regularly with a nutritionist and a psychologist. She was on her way to recovering from the early stages of the female athlete triad. Janice's recovery is ongoing—not a one-shot deal. She'll need to adopt a new outlook on her life in general, and apply it every day, to truly free herself from the syndrome.

You may plan to touch base with the person again. You might offer to share some reading material with her or let her know that she can talk to you any time if she ever feels like it. Keep the communication lines open. If you know that she has medical problems or amenorrhea, or if her conversation reveals a negative self-image, be prepared to suggest that she see a medical doctor for a checkup or a psychologist to help her with body image or self-esteem issues. You can offer to go with her. By raising your concerns with her, you may be helping her start the long journey to recovery. Your concern may save her life.

One night, **Angie** heard **Kathy** running in her room. She knocked and went in. She asked Kathy what she was doing. Kathy told her it was her new exercise program. Angie could see how thin Kathy was and how her bones stuck out, and she became even more worried. Angie had done enough reading and had prepared herself to talk again with Kathy. She said, "I just wanted to touch base with you, and see how things are going. I'm worried about you because you seem so moody, and you're losing a lot of weight." Kathy said that she was fine, and that she was finally getting into shape. Angie repeated that she was worried about her, not only because she was losing so much weight but also because she was not having her periods. Angie asked her if she would be willing to read some things that she had just come across about a newly discovered syndrome called the female athlete triad. Kathy had not heard about it and said she would.

A few nights later, Angie talked to Kathy again. Angie asked if she had read the brochure about the triad and if she had any questions. Kathy told her that she thought the triad was just for Olympic-type athletes. She said that all the girls on the swim team were dieting to make weight and were happy when they didn't get their periods. It seemed perfectly normal to her! Angie told her that it wasn't really normal to miss her period and that maybe she should go in for a checkup. Angie offered to go with her for her examination. Angie again said she brought this up only because she was concerned about her and loved her. Kathy saw that Angie was ready to cry and that she did not seem jealous, but really worried. Angie's worry did something to Kathy. She did not really know what it was, but something seemed to click inside. Somewhat reluctantly, Kathy gave up fighting against Angie and agreed to go with her for a gynecological checkup. She rationalized to herself that she needed to go anyway, and how bad could it be? Angie was really relieved.

What You Can Do to Help

◆ Be informed. Check into reading material and resources who can provide treatment. (See the resources section.)

◆ Be prepared. Have reading material and referrals to medical professionals ready, and offer to go with her for help.

- Talk to her with consistent, caring concern.
- Avoid judging, threatening, accusing, analyzing, or second guessing.
- Be honest.
- Talk to her in a private place when you are not pressured for time. Assure her of confidentiality.
- Use "I" statements, reflecting your honest concerns and observations.
- Expect denial, shame, embarrassment, or fear.
- If she denies or refuses help, try again.
- In the meantime, do not change your eating habits around her.
- Do not talk to others about her behind her back.
- If you have concerns about her immediate health or safety, tell her how worried you are and request to talk to her parents or significant other.
- Don't be mislead or deceived by her denial. Continue to approach her.
- Do not scrutinize or chide her for the food choices she does make when eating. This is not something to bring up over a meal in the dining hall.

FORMING YOUR SUPPORT TEAM

There is no one right type of help. Just as the women affected by the female athlete triad vary in their experiences, as is clear from the scenarios involving Hannah, Janice, Kathy, and Angie, each woman is different and has different needs. Treatment needs to be tailored to these individual needs and situations.

Start with one professional, usually a medical doctor, who can help you arrange any needed referrals to other professionals. As in athletics, each member of the team brings a certain skill, experience, and knowledge to the treatment plan. The core team consists of a medical care provider, a mental health provider, and a nutritionist. Other professionals may be needed as consultants, depending on your particular situation. A dentist may need to help you if you have dental damage from bulimia. A cardiologist (a doctor who specializes in disorders of the heart) may be called upon if you have heart problems. One of the professionals on the team will be the leader and will coordinate the care and the advice. Think of that person as your advocate, as the person with whom you touch base if things seem too confusing, out of control, or frightening. If your team leader is a sports medicine specialist, she can help you get back to your previous level of activity and then reach new heights of performance.

Core Members of the Treatment Team

A core member of your treatment team is the professional who provides medical care. She will do the physical examination, order tests, treat medical problems, arrange referrals, and decide about physical activity. The medical care provider can be a physician from the field of pediatrics, internal medicine, family medicine, sports medicine, or adolescent medicine, or she can be a nurse practitioner or physician's assistant. This person should have training and experience in treating the disorders of the female athlete triad and should be willing to work with other professionals, with your family, and with friends if indicated. If you are an athlete, she should understand the importance of your sport or physical activity in your life, and she should work closely with your coaches, trainers, and athletic administrators.

Another key member of the team is a mental health care provider. She may be a licensed psychologist (PhD); a psychiatrist (MD); a marriage, family, and child counselor (MFCC); or a licensed clinical social worker (LCSW). This person should have training and experience in working with active, athletic women and dealing with eating disorders and the female athlete triad. She will work with you on the psychological aspects of the triad, including your body image and stress management, and she will establish a specific treatment tailored to your needs. If you are significantly depressed or suicidal, she may advise hospitalization. If medication is considered as part of your treatment, you will need to see a professional who can prescribe it, usually a psychiatrist. Group or family therapy may also be part of your treatment plan.

Most women with the female athlete triad benefit from consulting with a nutritionist. Nutritionists are most often licensed as registered dietitians (RDs) and some may have other degrees as well, such as a master's in public health (MPH) or a PhD. She will help you establish a basic food program so you can meet your daily needs for protein, calcium, and other essential nutrients. She can help you design food plans and deal with difficult eating situations. You may find she gives you permission to eat foods that you once thought were forbidden, and she will help you reestablish a normal eating

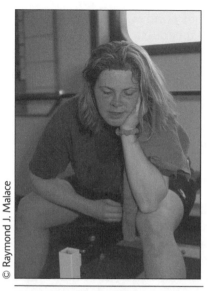

© Raymond J. Malace

Each member of your treatment team should inspire your trust.

pattern. In most cases, food and issues about eating are not the core problems, but rather the symptoms of underlying psychological issues. The dietitian's goal is not to force you to eat or to gain weight, but to get you to nourish your body and brain so you can perform and feel better in all that you do. She can educate you about nutrition and help you put what you learn into practice. She will help you address fears and misconceptions about food and enable you to return to balance in what you eat.

How do you know if the person you are seeing has the right training, experience, or credentials? If you are unsure, ask! Trained and experienced professionals are proud of their training and degrees and will be glad to explain them to you. They should be up front about their experience with the female athlete triad disorders and offer to give you names of other clients who have given their permission to be contacted. In addition to the training and the degree a professional has, it is important that she inspire your trust and confidence. You should be able to talk openly with her about your feelings as well as about any medical or psychological problems. If you have been forced into treatment, it may take a while to develop a trusting relationship. In that situation, the professional will need to establish a connection with you. She should understand your feelings, whether they are denial, anger, fear, embarrassment, or desperation. The right fit between you and your principal care providers is an important requirement if you are to make progress. If you do not feel comfortable with one person, do not give up treatment. Seek another referral until you find someone with whom you are comfortable working.

Other Treatment Team Members

If you are on an athletic team, your care providers may need to communicate with the trainer, coach, assistant coaches, and athletic administrators. These people will not be part of your treatment but may be involved in managing your training and competition status on a day-to-day basis. How they are involved will be determined by several factors.

Most important are your health and safety and your right to privacy. Your doctor or psychologist will ask for your permission to release any information to the athletic team staff (see page 218) for more about confidentiality). Their involvement should be supportive and helpful to you. A meeting between your doctors and the team staff can help determine guidelines for their involvement. They may be instructed not to weigh you, to ensure that you are treated as a full member of the team, and to leave any decision about participation to the medical care provider. Because of their roles in training the team, they will need to know any training restrictions you have.

GETTING REFERRALS

If you are ready, willing, and able to get treatment, start with the medical professional who knows you best. That might be your family doctor or nurse, or a team physician. They usually know the best resources in your community and can help with the first appointment and other referrals. If you are on a team, the athletic trainers are excellent referral sources. Most likely they have known other athletes with similar problems and have developed a referral network in the area. School nurses, nutritionists, and personal trainers may also have good referral sources from helping other clients.

Often the best referrals come from people who have gone through treatment themselves. You may know someone who has had an eating disorder and perhaps has dealt with all three of the triad conditions. She may suggest some of the best people in your area to see. You can call the local college or university health service for community referrals. If you are enrolled in school, many student health services have treatment plans on campus. Your local hospital and mental health center may also have referral lists. Most institutions will give you three or more names and let you decide who suits you the best. If you cannot identify a local resource, there are several national organizations that can help you with referrals. See the resources section for the contacts for the American College of Sports Medicine (ACSM), Anorexia Nervosa and Related Eating Disorders, Inc. (ANRED), and the National Association of Anorexia Nervosa and Associated Disorders (ANAD). The Internet can also be a source of information about referrals. Several Web sites are specific to the female athlete triad, and there are others devoted to eating disorders. If you use the Internet, be aware that not all services or referrals have been screened by professional organizations.

What to Look for in a Professional

Find a professional who

- ◆ is licensed and trained in his or her field (i.e., has the correct degree from a reputable institution),
- ◆ has specific training and experience in the triad disorders,
- ◆ is willing to work with you as part of a team of professionals,
- ◆ develops a sense of trust with you,
- ◆ ensures confidentiality,
- ◆ (if you are an athlete), understands the sport environment and is willing to work with the people affiliated with your athletic team, and
- ◆ works with you on helping arrange payment for services, either with your insurance, medical plan, or self-payment.

Angie and **Kathy** went together to see the primary care sports medicine doctor who had covered some of their swim meets in high school. Kathy tried to cancel at the last minute, but Angie would not let her. It was Angie's support that helped her walk in the door. The doctor asked Kathy what she could help her with. Kathy said that Angie had made her come because she wasn't having her period, and it was time for her checkup anyway. After a few more questions, the doctor asked Angie to leave, and she talked to Kathy alone.

The doctor remembered Kathy from the high school swim team and was surprised at how thin she had become in the past year. She recognized at once that Kathy had the signs of the female athlete triad. She knew how hard it had been for Kathy to come in, and she gently asked her how she was feeling. Kathy blurted out that she didn't want to be forced to have her period or gain weight. The doctor said she understood. She asked Kathy about how the first year at college had gone. Kathy said everything was great and that she was finally getting into shape. She admitted her grades had not been too good and that a lot of the time she felt out of the sorority scene. She said her only problems were feeling tired a lot and getting pressure from her family to gain weight. The doctor asked if she had lost a lot of weight and how she did it. Kathy proudly claimed to have lost 23 pounds since starting college. Her doctor then talked about her energy balance and showed her the energy equation (see chapter 5). Together they calculated that Kathy was in a state of energy imbalance. No wonder she was tired all the time! The doctor also let Kathy know that not having a menstrual period was not a normal sign of getting into shape but rather a sign of something going wrong. She gave Kathy a pamphlet describing the female athlete triad.

She congratulated Kathy for coming in for help and asked her if she agreed with the goals of recovering her energy and preventing any damage to the bones or to her overall health caused by not having her period. They agreed that Kathy wanted to have more energy and improve her performance on the swim team. The doctor recommended that Kathy meet with a nutritionist to plan what Kathy could eat comfortably. She also suggested she see a sport psychologist. In the meantime, she asked her to stop her rigorous training because of her irregular heartbeats. She also advised her to increase her calcium intake. Finally, the doctor ordered a few tests to check her heart and her bone density and to assess the cause of her amenorrhea. She told Kathy to call if she had any questions and to return in a week for a complete physical and to get the results of her tests.

Kathy felt relieved that she wasn't going to be forced to gain weight and told Angie that it hadn't been as bad as she had thought it would be. Angie offered to go with her to the other appointments and to look up some more information about the female athlete triad on the Internet. They went out for a frozen yogurt together. Angie felt somewhat hopeful that Kathy would return to normal now that she was going to get treatment.

What About Support Groups?

Support groups can also be part of treatment. Many offer an accepting environment of people who have gone through some of the same struggles as you and who can give you perspective, support, encouragement, and help. Most of us know about the successful 12-step programs central to alcoholic recovery like Alcoholics Anonymous (AA). A similar program has been developed called Overeaters Anonymous (OA). Many patients with bulimia and many binge overeaters have found help in these groups. It's important to know that according to guidelines issued by the American Psychiatric Association, 12-step programs are not recommended as the first or the only treatment approach; however, they may be very useful as additional support to regular psychological therapy.

In addition to 12-step programs, there are other types of support groups that might be useful for someone recovering from the female athlete triad disorders. Most focus on the issues of disordered eating. For example, people who have been in group psychological therapy may form a support group after formalized group therapy ends. These follow-up groups can affiliate with a mental health professional who provides advice and guidance. In addition, many high school and college campuses have peer-led support groups that focus on body image, weight issues, nutrition, or eating disorders. Local chapters of national eating disorder organizations also have support groups. Churches or other religious organizations may have support groups, Bible study classes, or professionally led groups that focus on self-esteem or disordered eating. Some athletic teams form peer-led support groups. There is a great deal of variation from group to group. Your mental health therapist can help you assess the group and whether or not it is right for you. Check with him or her before joining a support group. And then you may want to try several until you find one that matches your needs and interests.

Will My Medical Insurance Pay for Treatment?

Before you go for treatment, check what type of medical coverage and insurance you have, and call your insurance provider to find out what is covered. Check your coverage before you seek medical care, or the medical services may not be paid for by the insurance company. Certain services and tests may not be part of your medical plan. For example, blood tests to evaluate amenorrhea may be covered by your plan, but a bone density test may not. If you and your physician feel that you need a particular test that your plan does not cover, you may be able to write an appeal to your insurance carrier. If you are not covered, do not let this stop you from getting treatment. Getting treatment for the triad disorders as soon as possible will help you regain your health and energy sooner, will minimize long-term damage to your body, and will allow you to achieve your peak health and fitness faster.

When **Kathy** went back for a follow-up visit, the sports medicine doctor told her that the tests indicated she had low levels of estrogen and had lost bone mass. She had the female athlete triad, and her doctor was concerned about heart damage from the starvation diet and overexercise. Kathy had read enough to understand about the triad and asked the doctor her most worrying questions. Would she have to give up swimming and gain a lot of weight? The doctor reassured her that she would not have to, but that recovery from the triad meant working with several other specialists and would take time.

Kathy gave the doctor permission to speak with her nutritionist and psychologist to work out a treatment plan. Kathy wasn't sure what to tell her parents, coach, and friends. The doctor suggested that Kathy be honest and tell them what had been going on. They could call her office and she would inform them about Kathy's needs. A few days later, Kathy's mother admitted that she knew something was seriously wrong with Kathy, but she did not know what to do about it. Kathy and her mother went to see the doctor together. The doctor said that Kathy would need several months or more of treatment and that much of the treatment would be with a psychologist.

Kathy's parents talked to her about getting treatment at home or going back to school. The doctor suggested that some of treatment would be family therapy. Kathy agreed that she should stay home from school for one year. They contacted her college coach and the administration to arrange a leave of absence. Angie felt an enormous sense of relief. Her sister was going to get help and hopefully get better.

MAKING THE JOURNEY TO RECOVERY

With the professionals on your treatment team, you will set goals and priorities for treatment. Think of the treatment plan as a road map on your journey to recovery. Before you start any road trip, the vehicle, in this case your body, must be in good working order. So the first part of the treatment is a checkup of your physical and mental health. Are there any immediate risks to your life that would require you to be in a hospital or on medication? Are you seriously depressed or suicidal and in need of intensive psychological help? Are your electrolytes out of balance and in need of a tune-up? What do you need to know to take this journey? Who should be on the trip with you?

Hospitalization

The first priority is to make sure you do not have a serious medical or psychological problem that needs to be treated in the hospital (see the following list). If you do, you need to be treated and stabilized before determining long-term treatment plans. Examples of serious medical problems requiring hospitalization include the following:

- ◆ Significant weight loss—20 percent or more below healthy body weight and failure to maintain or gain weight as an outpatient—which is associated with damage to the heart, kidneys, or brain

- ◆ Inability to control bingeing and purging to the extent that few other activities are possible

- ◆ Serious metabolic problems, such as a low potassium or acid/base disorder, that require intravenous treatment

- ◆ Symptoms of cardiac abnormality, such as irregular heartbeats

- ◆ Passing out or fainting

- ◆ Significant abnormality on the EKG (electrocardiogram)

- ◆ Suicidal intent

- ◆ Serious bone fracture that requires surgery and hospitalization to stabilize

Contracts and Releases of Information

If you do not have a life-threatening problem, you will start seeing your care providers for outpatient treatment. The first order of treatment is to establish treatment goals and priorities. If you are on an athletic team, you will also need to establish guidelines for participation. If you are not in an organized team program, consult with your doctor about your training or activity. Sometimes the treatment goals and the participation plan are written up in a treatment contract that you will sign. Your care providers may also start a treatment sheet that helps them monitor your goals and your progress toward them.

Your doctors will also review your consent to treatment and authorization for release of information. If you are under 18 years of age, your parent or guardian needs to provide consent and authorization for your treatment. If you are over 18 years old, you alone have the right to consent to treatment and to authorize the release of information about your care. Very strict laws regulate the release of medical information so that your confidentiality is protected. No aspects of your treatment or records can be released to anyone without your consent. This means that if you are over 18 no one, including your parents, coach, employer, or professors, can see your medical records without your written consent. If someone needs to see your records, such as a consulting physician or an insurance company, you must sign a statement releasing the information only to the people you designate. Before members of your treatment team can even speak to each other about you, you have to give them consent to do so. Make sure you review and understand what you are consenting to. If you are uncertain, ask questions.

Fears About Treatment

The first question and greatest fear many women have about treatment is, "Am I going to get fat?" Many are more concerned about gaining weight than about the medical and psychological problems they are battling with the triad disorders. We've already learned (see chapters 1 through 4) that the fear of being fat can lead to eating disorders and thus to the triad. It is why many women do not want treatment. If this "fat fear" is keeping you from seeking help, you should know that the goal of your treatment is definitely not to make you fat. The treatment goals are ultimately set for you to recover your mental and physical health, restore your energy balance, improve your athletic performance, and develop a positive sense of self and body image. If you are undernourished, gaining some weight might be a necessary consequence of recovering your health. If you gain weight in treatment, most of the weight gain should be muscle as you begin to supply your body with the energy it needs to go from too thin to win to too fit to quit.

If you think about it, there really is no way that someone else can make you fat. If you have an eating disorder, you may fear becoming overweight or feeling fat, but in reality you are usually underweight or normal weight. Your body image is the problem. Fat fears are often signs of fear about other issues, such as not being liked, not being perfect, not being in control, not being attractive, or not being good enough. These fears and feelings can best be addressed and solved in psychological treatment.

Another part of treatment is learning to properly nourish your body instead of starving it and then overeating later in desperation. People who eat normally and avoid the overeating that comes with dieting achieve and remain at a body weight that is healthy for them. Remaining physically active during treatment is another reason you will not gain too much weight.

Perhaps you say that you know someone who was treated for anorexia and now she is really fat? It can happen, but it is an indication that her treatment was incomplete or not successful. The people who become very overweight have not addressed and solved their underlying problems. They continue to use food as a method to treat stress, depression, low self-esteem, or anxiety. If you stay in treatment and work through your underlying issues, then you will not get fat. Instead, you will have a normal body weight, a healthy self and body image, and improved athletic performance.

The Treatment Plan

So, just what will happen with treatment? Which map should you follow for your trip? Because everyone is different, there is no one specific treatment plan or length of treatment. A great deal will depend on you—on where you want and need to go. How many stops do you need along the way?

To start the trip, discuss your desired destination with your treatment team so they can design the best route. They should know your goals, both for your performance and for personal success. If you are starting therapy, start by listing your goals in these areas and discussing them with your therapist. You can also help your therapist by identifying what your problem areas are—is it your family, your schoolwork, your relationships, your training, or trying to balance them all?

If you are contemplating entering treatment or are in treatment, stop here for a moment and write down your goals. Openly discuss them with your health care providers and see if they are on the same path. Your goals may not be identical to theirs, but the goals should be similar and all of them should focus on your well-being. If you are concerned that your health care providers are trying to make you "fat," discuss that out in the open. If there are parts of your life that you are not ready or willing to work on, let them know that, too.

Part of your complete recovery will involve working with the nutritionist to plan the fuel for your journey. You need to know how to meet your basic needs for daily life, how often to stop for fuel, and what fuel additives you might need. By fuel additives, we mean vitamin and mineral supplements, especially iron supplements (if you are anemic) and calcium supplements (if you are unable to get enough calcium in your diet; see table 6.3).

The medical doctor will work with you to correct any medical problems so that you do not break down and need repairs on this trip. If you have amenorrhea, your doctor will find out why and treat you so that your menstrual cycles resume (see chapter 5). If you have osteoporosis, hormone replacement or other bone-building therapies (see chapter 6) may be prescribed.

A big part of your treatment is the care provided by the mental health practitioner. Think of her as the mapmaker and guide who makes sure you are on the right path and helps you get back on track if you go astray. You need to check in frequently, because some of the territory you are traveling in is largely unmapped and is new to you. In the beginning of treatment, your therapist will touch base with you and see what your motivation for treatment is. Do you recognize a problem and want to solve it? Or do you feel you are being forced into treatment? What is going on in your journey through life? Are there mountains to climb or rivers to cross? Do you have the right tools to do this? Are there struggles with coaches or family members, at work or school, or in relationships? How do you feel about yourself and your body?

It is helpful to identify the sources of stress in your life. Eating disorders are often a coping mechanism for stress, depression, anxiety, or other emotional problems. If bingeing and purging occur when you are under stress, you will learn other ways to deal with stress. If you feel anxious around food, you can work with a therapist to be more comfortable in situations you cannot control. Together, you will work to understand the underlying factors that cause and perpetuate disordered eating behavior. Part of treatment is getting to know and like yourself better. Learning new, healthier coping mechanisms is a key part of treatment. These coping techniques will be useful for the rest of your life as you face other mountains and rivers.

Along with your medical doctor and your nutritionist, your therapist will help you be comfortable adopting a healthy eating plan and reversing your energy imbalance. Through individual or group therapy, you will work on correcting negative thoughts about yourself and improving your body image. Often you will be encouraged to keep a written journal of your journey. This is a tool for self-reflection, expression, and learning. Being able to express what you are feeling is part of learning about yourself and the factors that may be troubling you.

An important decision when you start therapy is whether to work in individual or group therapy, or both. Sometimes it is better to cross dangerous territory in the company of others who can provide support. That decision will be made with your mental health care provider. Family members may also be included in therapy, in which case the family, rather than the individual, is the focus of the therapy. Your therapist will also evaluate you for problems besides those of the female athlete triad. Frequently, other issues are involved with disordered eating behavior. They may include depression, anxiety, personality disorders (such as perfectionism and obsessive-compulsive disorder), alcohol or other substance abuse, sexual abuse, stealing and shoplifting, and self-destructive behavior such as self-mutilation. These issues will also need to be evaluated and treated.

Will you require medication? That depends on your individual situation and needs. Some antidepressants have been shown to be effective in reducing binge eating and managing depression. If you have particular trouble with those symptoms, medication may be prescribed. If any medication is considered at all, you should be fully informed of the reasons why, the side effects, and the duration of treatment. Most of these medications do not impair athletic performance, but you will want to check with your doctor to find out about any interactions or side effects.

Kathy, her psychologist, and her medical doctor each separately wrote out their goals. Kathy's goals were to stay thin, to be able to work out every day, and to not feel so tired. The doctor's goals were to make sure she had no underlying heart problems causing her racing heartbeat, to correct her energy imbalance, to restore normal body weight, to treat her amenorrhea, and to ensure that Kathy take in 1,500 mg of calcium a day. The psychologist's goals were to improve Kathy's self-image, to help her with her interpersonal relationships, and to get her to consider family therapy.

After discussing these goals with her doctors, Kathy understood that she felt tired because of her energy imbalance. She felt okay about working on a plan to get her energy back in balance. She agreed to eat some additional calcium-rich foods every day and to cut back her training until her heart tests were normal and she regained some energy. The doctor told her that weight was not the most important thing, but rather her overall health and sense of well-being. She pointed out that Kathy was weighing herself too often and obsessing about the number on the scale. The doctor asked her to get rid of the scale.

At first, Kathy was shocked and said no. Weighing herself was a big part of her life. How could she live without it? How would she know if she was fat or thin? How would she know how much she could allow herself to eat? After discussing the issues about the scale at two visits, Kathy finally agreed to move the scale out of her bathroom and into Angie's closet and to stop weighing herself. They agreed that if she felt too anxious, she could go back and use it. Otherwise, her weight would be monitored in the doctor's office. The doctor told Kathy to not look at the number on the scale, so Kathy turned her back when she was weighed in the doctor's office. As long as her weight was the same or had increased slightly, the doctor gave her the thumbs-up sign. At first, it felt strange, but after two weeks, Kathy experienced a sense of relief.

Kathy's heart tests turned out normal, and the doctor gave her medical clearance to begin working out again. She started stretching every day except Sunday, then slowly building up her exercise program with swimming, frequently checking her pulse.

Kathy found that the nutritionist was a really neat lady who had also been a swimmer in high school. They emphasized choosing foods Kathy liked to eat and not counting calories. To ensure 1,500 mg of calcium a day, Kathy blended a special smoothie, adding calcium powder, yogurt, and milk to her favorite fruit. Her homemade smoothies became very popular with her family.

With the psychologist, Kathy looked at pictures of herself in high school and photos of other swimmers and healthy, athletic women. Then they compared these with pictures of Kathy since her weight loss. Kathy could see she had lost her well-defined "swimmer's shoulders" and that she looked tired and not as fit as in the old pictures. Kathy had told the psychologist she was afraid of getting fat, but the pictures showed her that she never had been fat. She was reassured again that treatment goals were not to make her fat. She worked on thinking about food not as her enemy but as fuel for her body.

Kathy talked about her relationships with her family, their expectations, and how she handled the pressure of the first year at college by dieting. She admitted she did not like the chemistry class she had taken in the summer. With all the appointments and doctor's visits, Kathy sometimes felt overwhelmed, but Angie and her mother were always there to tell her that they loved her and would help her. Angie and Kathy's parents came to the psychologist for several sessions of family therapy, which helped the family understand Kathy's issues better.

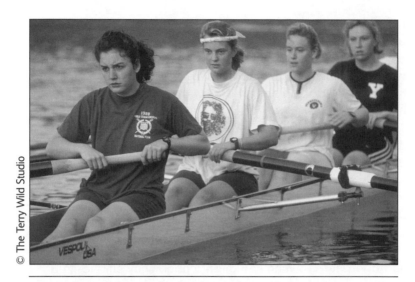

© The Terry Wild Studio

Medically approved exercise during recovery provides psychological and physical benefits.

Exercise During Treatment

Most likely, exercise is an important part of your life. It has numerous benefits, including reducing anxiety and depression, helping you feel healthy and in control, and maintaining cardiac fitness and bone mass. Part of your treatment plan will involve decisions about physical activity. The first goal is to keep you going in your current activities and training if it is medically safe to do so.

Your doctor will make sure there are no health risks associated with your exercise program. For some medical problems, you may need to modify or monitor activity. If you have a stress fracture, you will need to adjust your exercise until that injury heals. If you have abnormal electrolytes or an irregular heartbeat, you will not be able to exercise until these serious problems are corrected. If you have passed out at any time due to the triad, you need to be evaluated and treated before it is safe for you continue to exercise. After a complete evaluation, if you are medically cleared for exercise you may be referred to a monitored exercise program in which your heart rate and blood pressure are checked during your workouts. During treatment and recovery, your exercise program should help you, not put you at further risk for injury or a heart problem. It should not be overly strenuous. When you are taking a trip in a car, you check the oil and gas and drive at a safe speed. Same with exercise. Ensure that your gas and water tanks are full by getting enough food and water for your exercise.

The goal of your exercise program during treatment is to maintain your overall fitness while improving your energy balance. Your recovery exercise program should incorporate the general principles of any well-designed exercise program, including warm-up, stretching, cool-down, aerobic training, and strength training.

Warm-Up

The warm-up is the first part of any exercise session. Think about what your body is like before you start exercising. It is like a car that has been sitting outside on a cold day. It needs to be warmed up to get the oil flowing throughout the engine before it can perform at its best. Likewise, before you start exercising, most of the blood flow is directed at your heart, brain, kidneys, and digestive organs. You need to get the blood flowing to your muscles, tendons, and ligaments by doing some gentle exercise (like jumping rope, stationary bicycling, or jogging) until you start to break a sweat. That means blood flow has been redistributed to the skin and muscles and they are warm and ready to stretch.

Stretching

The purpose of stretching before and after exercise is to reduce injuries, increase the lubrication of joints, and decrease the formation of scarring or tight muscles from overuse. If you have been overtraining or have chronic injuries that do not heal, most likely you have many areas that are tight and inflexible. They need to be restored to function and balance before you can successfully exercise at moderate or high levels. You want to systematically stretch all the major muscle groups you use in your exercise and stretch around any injured joints or tendons. If you have injuries, check with your physician for the proper type of stretching and strengthening for your injury.

To stretch correctly, hold each stretch for a count of 10 to 30 while breathing slowly and relaxing into the stretch. You should feel a gentle stretch, not pain. Do not bounce up and down; that actually ends up tightening the muscles and can cause injury. Certain stretching programs, such as yoga and gentle, flowing exercise like tai chi, are very useful for flexibility and relaxation. If you have a stress or full fracture, are moderately malnourished, or have other medical problems, stretching can be an excellent form of exercise to do until you are able to resume your usual activity.

Aerobic Exercise

Aerobic exercise is the type of exercise that gets your heart going and your lungs and sweat glands pumping. Running, bicycling, brisk walking, aerobic dancing, and swimming for 15 to 60 minutes are examples of aerobic exercise. Aerobic exercise trains and conditions the heart, lungs, and circulatory system to work more efficiently, and it is linked to that great feeling known as runner's high.

Before resuming aerobic exercise, check with your doctor to determine your level of intensity and the length of time you should exercise. To ensure that you are in a safe and effective zone to get the most out of aerobic exercise, monitor your heart rate and compare it to the target heart rate zone described by your doctor. Keep in mind that to maintain your fitness, you need to do aerobic exercise only three to five times a week, not every day. Everyone needs at least one or two days off a week from exercise, including professional athletes.

If you are exercising every day, you are doing too much, especially during treatment. If your doctor clears you for exercise, make sure you fuel up for it. This means increasing your fluid intake so that you do not get dehydrated and eating enough calories to match what you use. If you do not fuel up, you will be running on empty and will not get the benefits. You may end up breaking down muscle tissue, overstressing your heart, and putting yourself at risk for injuries. Monitor all exercise sessions by checking your pulse frequently to make sure you are in the target zone and are not experiencing irregular heartbeats. If you have any medical symptoms, such as light-headedness, irregular heartbeats, nausea, or injuries, contact your doctor for a checkup and do not continue to exercise.

Strength Training

If you lifted weights before beginning treatment, you may want to continue if you are medically cleared to do so. Strength training has the benefits of increasing your muscle mass and helping maintain or build bone mass. Ideally, strength train on alternate days from your aerobic training, usually two to three times a week for 15 to 60 minutes. You should always warm up and stretch before lifting weights. A physical therapist, personal trainer, or strength coach can advise you on the right way to lift and the right types of machines or free weights to use. In general, target specific muscle groups and choose weights that train the muscles you wish to strengthen. It is especially important to train the muscles of the back, trunk, abdomen, lower legs, and upper arms for the bone-building effects. Lift an amount of weight that is comfortable for you without straining. Never hold your breath. Lift this comfortable weight for 10 repetitions, rest a few seconds, then repeat 10 more lifts of the same weight if desired, for a total of one to three sets. Using heavy weights and doing fewer repetitions can increase muscle size and strength, whereas using lighter weights and doing more repetitions can increase muscle tone, definition, and endurance. Be sure to stay well hydrated while lifting, and stop and contact your physician if you feel any dizziness, lightheadedness, irregular heartbeats, or pain.

Cool-Down

After an exercise session, no matter what type, it is very important that you take the time to cool down to allow your body to return to normal levels of exertion, readjust the circulation system, and relax and feel that runner's high. You worked hard; you deserve it! After you finish your exercise, gradually slow your pace and walk for 5 to 10 minutes, drink some more water or a sport drink, check your pulse to make sure it is returning to normal rates, and mentally check your body to make sure you don't feel anything unusual. If you have any dehydration, electrolyte, or heart problems, a cool-down is essential to allow the circulatory system to gradually readjust the distribution of blood flow from the muscles back to the heart, brain, and kidneys. If you stop too quickly, you may feel faint or even pass out.

To refuel your muscles with glycogen, take in 200 to 400 calories of complex carbohydrate within 30 to 90 minutes after finishing your exercise. Your body is programmed to absorb and store glycogen, the fuel for your next workout, most effectively in this window of time.

Monitoring Your Exercise Plan

You and your doctor will be evaluating the safety and the effectiveness of your exercise plan as you go through treatment. Keep an exercise log for each day you work out, and take that in when you see your physician (see table 7.1). If you feel or notice anything unusual during your exercise, check with your doctor before exercising the next day.

CONTINUING TO TRAIN AND COMPETE

If it is safe and healthy for you to train and compete, and you still want to, the answer to your question is a qualified yes. You need to be under the care of a physician to make sure you are not at risk for injury or a cardiac problem from training or competing. You need to take responsibility for monitoring yourself during training and making sure you can keep up your nutrition and fluid intake to meet your training needs.

Table 7.1

Training Diary

Day	Monday	Tuesday	Wednesday
Resting pulse (before arising)			
Sleep hours			
Training pulse (maximum during training)			
Fluid intake			
Diet and caloric intake			
Mood			
Any injuries			
Aerobic training			
Strength training			
Other			

Note: If your resting pulse increases by 10 percent or more or if you have an injury that does not
Use the diet, sleep, fluid intake, and mood sections to see what you can improve in your training

Thursday	Friday	Saturday	Sunday

heal for 2 or more days, take a day off or reduce training.
and lifestyle if you're feeling tired or are injured.

Continuing in sport may have advantages for your treatment. You may be more motivated to get treatment if you can safely continue doing what you love to do while becoming fit and strong enough to do it well again. And treatment is likely to help your sport performance. Why? Because the female athlete triad is usually a state of energy imbalance and impaired performance. Getting treatment can reduce your risk of injury, restore your energy balance, and fuel your body so that you can train and compete even better than before. The more positives that are associated with getting treatment, the more likely you are to stay in treatment and to benefit from it. Staying in training and competition can give you a sense of well-being, self-esteem, and identity. You are more likely to do well in treatment if you are in your normal environment. If you continue your sport while you are in treatment, you can take what you learn back to your sport and continue to participate in a healthy way.

How can you and your family, trainer, and coaches decide if you can stay in sport while you get treatment? If you are an athlete in a college or high school sport, it will be the responsibility of the team physician to decide on your status for participation. If you are not on a team, it will be up to the physician on your treatment team to make the decision.

Requirements for a Woman With the Triad to Participate in Sport and Exercise

- ❖ You are under the care of a physician or a treatment team monitoring your medical and psychological status.
- ❖ You are keeping your appointments with the treatment team.
- ❖ If necessary, you have signed a treatment contract and are adhering to it.
- ❖ If there is a change in your condition (such as an injury or illness), you will be reevaluated for sport participation.
- ❖ Training sessions are monitored and may be reduced in the interest of your medical safety. Monitoring can include checking pulse and hydration status and eliminating certain parts of the training.
- ❖ In general, for training and competition you should be at no less than 90 percent of your healthy body weight.
- ❖ You are eating and drinking appropriately for your sport.
- ❖ You are not losing more than a half-pound a week. Ideally, your weight is stable or you are gaining weight if needed.
- ❖ You have no other illness or injuries that would take you out of training or competition.
- ❖ You genuinely want to train and compete.

Most women want to continue in their sport or exercise and should be allowed to do so while they are being treated for the triad disorders. However, there are several situations in which it is best for your health and well-being to stop your sport or physical activity for awhile in order to recharge your battery and get a new perspective.

Reasons to Stop Sport or Physical Activity During Treatment

- You are at risk for a serious medical problem such as a fracture, heart problems, fainting, or kidney failure.
- You do not want to stay in the sport and are doing it for someone else or for some other reason.
- The sport environment perpetuates the triad disorders.
- You are suicidal or severely depressed.
- The sport environment conflicts with treatment and makes treatment impossible.
- You have injuries that do not heal.
- Your continuing participation on the team adversely affects the rest of the team.

Certainly the main reason to stop is that you are at serious medical or psychological risk. Having the triad is bad enough, but you do not want to develop other problems, such as a fractured bone or heart failure. If you are participating in a sport that you are not enjoying or feel you are doing it for someone else, then you need to stop and reevaluate your participation for awhile. If the sport or the training situation is reinforcing behavior that is damaging your body, you will not get well until you take a break from the sport. For example, if you participate in a sport that requires frequent weigh-ins, and you cannot make that weight without disordered eating behavior, you need to step back from the sport. Or if you participate in ballet or aerobics, where you constantly see yourself in front of a mirror and compare yourself to others, you may need to take yourself out of that environment for awhile. If you are in a debilitated state, your continued participation on a team may disrupt the team and affect your teammates' performance as well. For example, if you are a gymnast with bulimia, and you pass out or fall off an apparatus, your coach and teammates may feel they cannot rely on you in an upcoming competition.

It is up to you and your treatment team to evaluate your situation. Here are some questions to help you determine whether or not you should continue in your sport or physical activity.

◆ Is sport part of your problem, particularly if it is an activity like gymnastics, ballet, or diving, where any weight gain may be a problem?

◆ Is the intense competition and stress of the sport part of your emotional stress?

◆ Does the sport reinforce the female athlete triad disorders and make it likely that you will not be successful in the treatment or further prevention of these disorders?

◆ Are you malnourished or osteoporotic and therefore at risk for a fracture or injury?

◆ Are you training intensively with injuries that do not heal?

◆ Do you have serious medical problems, such as fainting, that are likely to cause problems?

◆ Do you understand the medical and psychological risks you face and the reasons your family, friends, and so many professionals are concerned about you?

Consider reviewing these questions and your answers to them with your treatment team to work out the best solution.

Kathy stopped swimming for a while because of her exercise-associated rapid heartbeat. Although her heart tests were normal, her rapid heartbeat was a sign of overtraining, dehydration, and exhaustion. She was able to get 1,500 mg of calcium a day and was doing some stretching and light weight lifting. Her doctor had her increase her fluids and calories. She taught her to monitor her pulse at rest and during weight lifting and told her to keep it under 120 beats per minute. After that, Kathy did not have the symptoms of a racing heart anymore. Two months later, she had more energy and was happy with the muscle tone in her arms she saw from lifting weights. Her weight had increased five pounds, most of it muscle, and she resumed her periods. She was cleared to start swimming again, with frequent pulse checks.

During her recovery at home, Kathy did not miss the people from college and started hanging out with a few high school friends who were taking classes at the local junior college. She told her friends at college that she was taking a year off to decide what she wanted to major in and to get her grades up. She did not feel ready to tell friends and others that she had the female athlete triad, and no one pressed her for more information. She kept a daily journal of her feelings and moods and found that she frequently felt anxious and inadequate. She hated chemistry and did not know what she wanted to be when she got out of college. She wasn't sure that being a doctor or a lawyer was for her. She was able to discuss these feelings with the psychologist.

In family therapy, they set ground rules for dealing with Kathy's eating and weight. As long as Kathy kept appointments with the treatment team, her parents and Angie would not discuss her diet or weight. Kathy told her parents about how much pressure she felt to be the best at everything. Her parents worked on letting Kathy know they loved her no matter what she was doing. When she felt anxious, Kathy wrote down what was bothering her and worked out ways of dealing with it with the psychologist. They both agreed that Kathy enjoyed seeing friends, and she started calling friends up to go out. She even ate pizza with a group after going to a movie. Angie was back at school, 500 miles away, but she stayed in touch with Kathy every day by e-mail, sending her funny cartoons and stories she thought would cheer her up.

TALKING TO FRIENDS, FAMILY, AND COACHES

One of the most difficult things about the recovering from the triad is that it can be embarrassing to admit you have these disorders and if you are in treatment, what to tell others can be a dilemma. You may not want anyone associated with your sport or work to know that you are getting treatment. If a boss, family member, coworker, coach, or trainer wants to know about your treatment, usually it is because they are concerned about you. But you do not have to answer, as long as you are not seriously ill and missing work or workouts. Again, with the rules of confidentiality, your treatment is private.

If you want some information released, put in writing all agreements about the information to be released and who is allowed to receive it. Part of this release agreement should be that you have the right to change it at any time. If you are on an athletic team, the appropriate information to release to coaches and parents is that you are keeping appointments and are medically and psychologically cleared for participation. With the athlete's consent and in her presence, I have met with family members, teammates, and coaches. This has been helpful to all persons concerned as they struggle for guidelines and ground rules on how to deal with the triad disorders. It is a chance to educate and bring all supportive forces together to help you solve this complex problem. For women not on athletic teams, release of information to others is usually not necessary. However, it may be helpful to inform significant others in your life that you are following through with treatment.

> After the initial prodding by **Hannah**, **Janice** started seeing a psychologist and a nutritionist. She saw me for a complete medical checkup, and she agreed to increase her fluids to prevent the dehydration caused by her frequent vomiting. She scheduled her other appointments at times when she was not teaching, so did not have to tell her principal. A very private person, Janice didn't want her parents or her friends to know she was being treated for bulimia. She continued to go to the gym with Hannah and to a club on weekends with their friends. Hannah asked Janice how she was doing, and Janice told her things were going better, but that she preferred not to talk about it. This was fine with Hannah, because she could see that Janice was seeking help and making progress. Hannah decided she would just be Janice's friend and leave the treatment to the team of professionals. Six months later, at work, Janice showed Hannah a lesson plan on eating disorders she planned to present in one of her classes. Janice told Hannah she had learned a lot about eating disorders and thanked Hannah for helping her get treatment.

Talking to Teammates and Friends

Deciding what to say to teammates and friends can be difficult. Consult with your treatment team to determine what you want to say, not what you think your friends want to know. Think of it this way: if you were injured or had an illness like mononucleosis, you would see the team doctor to be checked and referred for treatment. You would not be practicing and competing until you were better. If teammates want to know why you aren't competing, you can handle it the same way you would handle any other illness or injury. You have a right to privacy and confidentiality.

Often your family, teammates, and friends are aware that something is going on with you. As in the cases of Kathy and Hannah, they may have urged you to get help, or you may have discussed certain

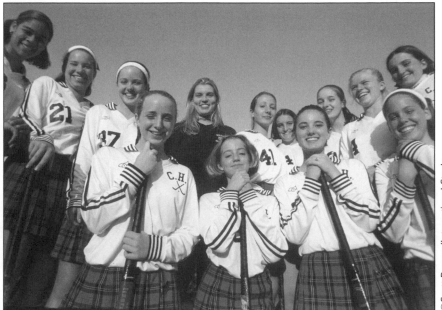

Teammates can be told as much or as little about your condition as you are comfortable with. They may be a great source of support.

aspects of the triad disorders with them. If you are comfortable being honest, that is the best policy. You do not have to tell everything; only what you are comfortable with. For example, you might say you just learned that not having menstrual cycles is a problem and that you are getting checked. Or you could say that you have been having problems with your diet and you are getting advice from a nutritionist. You could say that you are seeing a sport psychologist for help with stress management and sport performance. You could also say that you just learned about the dangers of the triad and are taking steps to get over it. Your honesty and willingness to talk can educate others and steer them to treatment as well. You may find that admitting to getting help is a great relief. No one is perfect. Intellectually, we all know that, but sometimes it is hard to admit. We are all human beings with flaws. We are bound to disappoint and displease others. Admitting that you are human is not such a bad thing and may even free more of your energy for other parts of life.

Dealing With Parents

If you are under 18, you will need your parents' (or guardian's) consent for treatment and possibly their help. If you are over 18, you can get treatment without parental consent. You may or may not want your parents to know about your problems and treatment. That is your right. Again, therapists cannot release information, even to your parents, without your consent unless there is an immediate risk to your life. Relationships with parents vary a great deal and the confidentiality issue needs to be individualized for your situation. Decisions about what to say to parents should be discussed with your treatment team. Part of your treatment may involve dealing with issues about your parents and family. Family therapy may be part of the treatment plan. Discuss with your therapist early in the course of treatment how much to say to your family, and come to a decision that is helpful and therapeutic for you. Often, your parents intuitively know something is wrong and want to help, but they may not have the knowledge, skills, or perspective to know what is best.

I frequently work with women to help them come up with ground rules for their parents. They include things such as asking your family not to comment or ask about your weight. You can tell them you are seeing medical personnel for this. You may also request that they not discuss your diet, including how much or what you are eating. You can tell them you are seeing a nutritionist. Work with your treatment team to decide what ground rules are comfortable and appropriate for you and your interactions with family and friends. In my experience, setting up ground rules provides a great relief and help in your daily life. It also relieves your parents and friends of having to worry about and feel responsible for you. Instead, they can express love and support.

Dealing With Coaches

A coach can be the most dominant person in an athlete's life. The coach's influence can be positive or negative. With your treatment team, you need to decide how to involve the coach and make that involvement as positive as possible. You and your treatment team can assess how much your coach understands about the female athlete triad. The first place to start is with education.

Coaches want to do the best job they can. However, they may not have the knowledge or experience to deal with these complicated disorders. If your coach is male, he may not have the life experience or sensitivity to understand the cultural pressures on women to be thin. A coach may place unreasonable weight pressures on you and your teammates without realizing the damage it can do. If you are going to stay on the team, you have to continue interacting with the coach. In my experience, many athletes are willing to have the coach involved in some manner. They want evidence of the coach's concern. Others are afraid the coach will kick them off the team or bench them. Every woman's situation is different, and dealing with the coach must be individualized.

There are certain situations where the coach's attitudes and training practices are harmful to the athlete. A coach who requires weigh-ins and then punishes athletes who do not make the weight can precipitate or exacerbate eating disorders. A coach who insists that amenorrhea is a healthy state for training and tells you not to take replacement hormones may be setting you up for osteoporosis. Training with an abusive or harassing coach is not worth it. These situations may require the athlete to leave the coach's sphere of influence for her health and treatment.

FINISHING THE JOURNEY

How long will treatment take? When will you know that you have recovered from the female athlete triad? Just as there is no one route for treatment, there is no one stopping point on the journey to health. You and your treatment team will assess your route and your progress frequently. If you voluntarily went to treatment and had not been suffering from the triad disorders for long, you might need only a few months of treatment. On the other hand, if you were in denial about having the triad and continued to participate in a lifestyle that perpetuated the disorders, treatment might take a long time. Treatment might not be effective until you eliminate the forces causing the triad from your life.

Many women with the triad, like Kathy, know they are getting better when their periods return to normal and stay that way for six months. For others, the sign they are better is that their natural energy and interest in life returns. Some women struggling with self-esteem and body image issues find that they feel better physically but that the emotional storms and psychological problems continue. Women with anorexia report that they must guard against "anorectic thinking" for the rest of their lives. Women with bulimia find they are tempted to return to purging when they are under stress or after weight gain.

As we've emphasized throughout this book, the triad disorders are common, chronic, and complex. The road to recovery is a journey over hills and through valleys, with many twists in the road. Sometimes it seems there is no end to the difficult journey of recovery. Other times, when you have gained some insight or have overcome an obstacle that seemed insurmountable, you feel a sense of freedom, hope, and enjoyment. You spend more days enjoying life and fewer days struggling with yourself. You feel better about who you are and you are no longer controlled by demons that make you exercise twice a day and always skip dessert. You can go out for dinner without worry. You can handle stressful situations and know that these too will pass. You have opened Pandora's box and have conquered your fears of the demons that can haunt all of us. You are your best self, and you got there by your own hard work and the love and support of others.

Six months after she started in therapy with her treatment team, **Kathy** felt much different from the driven first-year college student who counted Cheerios. She gained some weight, increased her strength, and did not think she looked "fat." In fact, she felt proud to have her swimmer's shoulders back. Working out three times a week, she had not weighed herself for months. She was honest with her parents and respectfully told them when they were bugging her. She took classes at the local junior college in art and art history, subjects she enjoyed but her parents disdained as not being practical. She had a group of friends and was dating a former boyfriend again. He told her he had been really worried about her and had thought she might have cancer. Kathy was able to trust him enough to tell him she had the female athlete triad and was getting help. He told her he loved her no matter what her weight was.

Kathy felt she had her energy back, and she wasn't too surprised when her menstrual cycles started again. She saw her medical doctor every eight weeks and stopped seeing the nutritionist. She also stopped private therapy, but went to a group therapy session once a week. She looked at the pictures taken of her when she was so thin and unhappy. Was this person really her? Had this really happened? Yes, it had. But thanks to the love and support of her sister, her parents, and her treatment team, she was recovering. She knew herself better and liked herself more.

The following fall, she returned to the university with the additional credits she had earned at the junior college. At first she was uncomfortable trying out for the swim team again. But her teammates soon welcomed her back, and they looked at her as a leader. She was able to advise some of the other members of the team and her coach about the female athlete triad. She had solved the riddle of the female athlete triad and was going to be okay.

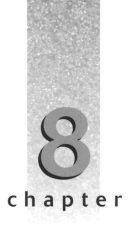

chapter

Peak Performance: Preventing the Triad

Having read the first seven chapters of this book, you no doubt are aware that the disorders of the female athlete triad are preventable. You also realize that they are often born of the current fad for thinness and nurtured by myths that to be successful, attractive, and happy, you must be thin—not just lean, but unrealistically thin, or too thin to win. As we've seen, this emphasis on thinness has not always been in vogue. In the 1960s, for example, free expression and rebellion against middle-class American values diminished the pressures and demands on women to be unrealistically thin. Bulimia was unknown. Women were still struggling for the right and the opportunity to be physically active and to play sports. The female athlete triad had not been recognized.

Young women grow up and experience the values of today's culture, but they are not as protected against the media blitz promoting thinness as women of the 1960s were. The young adult culture of the 1960s rejected judging a woman's worth by her weight. Today's culture glorifies thinness and makes it a prerequisite for being a fun, successful, and happy woman. Today, if you are not thin, you get the message that you should be unhappy. In the 60s, if you were not thin, you got the message to be yourself and to appreciate your natural body.

Our point is that culture influences our self-perception. Just as what is valued today is different from what was valued in the 1960s, there will continue to be many other cultural shifts with different icons for each one. The current ideal of the unrealistically thin woman is harmful to our health. If enough voices are raised so that strong, healthy women are celebrated in the media, then we will have a culture that helps instead of hurts women. Until there is a major shift in sociocultural norms, we must act at many levels to prevent women from developing the female athlete triad. Just as treatment involves a multidisciplinary team of professionals, prevention must be approached at many levels and by many different types of people.

WHAT YOU CAN DO

It is the individual who develops the triad, so most prevention plans should concentrate on decreasing individual risk factors. Genetic factors, such as a tendency toward depression or anorexia, cannot be changed. Other factors, such as being sexually abused or molested, are difficult (but not impossible) risk factors to change. Family dynamics and underlying personality disorders can be very difficult to modify. However, we can focus on the sociocultural, athletic, and developmental risk factors and provide women with the education and tools to stay healthy and fit.

Say No to Unrealistic Messages

We may not be able to change society in time to prevent the next generation from developing an unhealthy drive toward thinness and disordered eating, but through education, we can help women resist unrealistic messages. Although we have not been able to rid the world of certain illnesses, like mumps, measles, and chickenpox, vaccination programs prevent many people from getting these dreaded childhood diseases. Likewise, you can immunize yourself, your friends, your sisters, and your daughters against the assault of the message that "you can never be too thin."

Value Being Healthy, Fit, and Strong

To protect and inoculate yourself against society's harmful messages, it is most important to have a positive body image. Having a positive body image means accepting and loving the body you were born with. Develop the inner knowledge that your body is wonderful and that you are going to make the most of it. If you were not raised with a positive body image, do what you can to develop one now. Reject notions that you should look like someone else. Know what your best parts are and learn to accentuate them. If you have beautiful eyes, highlight them with makeup. Use a big smile to show off your beautiful teeth. You can keep a journal, learn visualization techniques, and work with a positive body image group or therapist. See chapter 1, pages 32 through 36 for more ideas and exercises for developing your positive body image.

How early should you hear these positive messages about your body? Most people say as early as age three or four. More positive messages should come around the time of puberty, when your body is changing so much. Part of a positive self-image includes choosing healthy role models. The women you admire should look more like you than like someone in a computer-enhanced photo. Where do you find appropriate role models? It might take some looking, but decide what you are looking for. You are likely to find pictures of more normal women in sports-related magazines like *Women's Sports and Fitness,* *Sports Illustrated for Women,* or *Jump* (for teens). Rent old movies featuring actresses with great individuality and strong personalities. Put up reprints of paintings and sculptures of beautiful women who are not prepubertal waifs. Seek out posters of athletic teams, like the ones at your local college, or of professional women tennis, softball, or basketball players. Support and learn about foundations like Melpomene, Women's Sports Foundation, and Women's Sport International. Look for photos of strong, athletic women like Karrie Webb or Sei Re Park (golf), Gabrielle Reece (volleyball), Lisa Leslie or Rebecca Lobo (basketball), Vanessa Atler (gymnastics), Lindsay Davenport, Martina Hingis, or Venus Williams (tennis), or the U.S. Women's soccer team members.

Celebrate your body and emphasize your good points. Make a list of your good points and accentuate the positive. Know how to de-emphasize your "bad" points, both physically and mentally. Stop looking at your thighs in the mirror every morning and obsessing about them. Choose clothing that de-emphasizes your thighs and highlights your strong arms. Or better yet, instead of battling your hips or thighs, choose to fight the ways women are unrealistically portrayed in the media. Write to an advertiser or a magazine editor and complain about the images of women you see in their products.

Concentrate on the things you do well, and work on improving your technique. Take care of your wonderful body, enjoy it, and create balance in your diet and exercise. Take classes in nutrition or

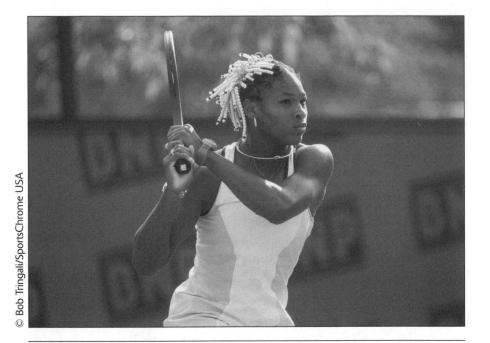

© Bob Tringali/SportsChrome USA

Serena Williams and other strong, powerful, and athletic women are positive role models.

read about the proper diet for your age and activity level. Take an exercise physiology class to learn the basics about healthy exercise and how the body functions. Learn how to monitor your heart rate to evaluate your training. Recognize when you have an injury and take care of it early. Follow the portion sizes and food choices recommended in the food pyramid. Take the calcium quiz (page 168), and ensure that you get enough calcium for your age and menstrual status. Make sure you get enough iron. Do your own energy equation, and stay in energy balance so you do not develop an energy drain. Eat when you are hungry, and enjoy eating after a hard workout. Do not be afraid of food. Give in to cravings and to the enjoyment of food.

Make a list of women and girls you admire, and notice that the main reason you admire your grandmother, or Madeline Albright, or Sandra Day O'Connor is not their appearance. If you only admire movie and television stars, broaden your horizons, and read about the history of women. Don't talk disparagingly about your weight or your body, particularly around younger girls. Young girls learn their own self-talk from others. You can influence not only your own self-talk but also that of friends and younger women by emphasizing positive things and de-emphasizing weight. Women can learn to love and accept their bodies if they see other women doing the same. How do you spend your money? Do you spend much of it on current fashions, diets, or makeup? And how much do you get out of it? Does the money you spend reflect your values, or those of advertisers? Spend some of that money in other areas. For instance, you might buy inspirational books about women or books on personal training, nutrition, or other topics that interest you. Or you could save for a special trip or experience.

A friend of ours once said, "If you believe reaching a certain weight goal is so important, try reading the obituaries and show me just once where it mentions 'reached ideal body weight' as a major accomplishment in someone's life."

Take the Disorder Out of Eating

The following are 12 ideas on how to prevent eating disorders. These ideas come from the book *Taking the Disorder Out of Eating* (1996) by Sarah Cates and Jennifer Steen. These women, while athletes and undergraduates at Duke University, formed peer groups to resist the messages that lead to disordered eating.

1. Tolerate diversity. Appreciate the variety of body shapes and sizes. Educate yourself about genetic as well as social bases of different weights.
2. Treat weightism just as seriously as racism, sexism, etc.
3. Be a critical consumer of both advertisement and social interaction.
4. Listen to internal cues of satiety and hunger.
5. Enjoy food.
6. Try eating without distractions such as televisions, studying, talking, or talking on the phone.
7. If you overeat, do not punish yourself with self-defeating thoughts, purging, or restriction.
8. Do not compare yourself to your peers. Everyone has different metabolisms, body shapes, and food preferences.
9. Reinforce normal eating among peers.
10. Recognize that females grow in adolescence and gain womanly curves.
11. Celebrate your body. Express yourself.
12. Love yourself.

Develop a Positive Self-Image

Positive self-image, or self-esteem, is another learned personality trait that will help you avoid the triad. There are many academic definitions and even different types of self-esteem. What we mean here is a feeling of self-worth. Basically, you feel good about yourself and no one else can change that feeling. You like yourself and what you do. You do things and dress a certain way because you like to, not because it is current fashion. Self-worth is established by parenting and by life experiences. If you were raised to be a perfectionist or were born with that personality trait, it is hard to have much self-esteem, because your expectations are always too high. However, if you set healthy, attainable goals and develop good self-esteem, you will not be as vulnerable to the swings and sways of fashion. You will not judge yourself harshly by external values, and you can stop self-destructive behaviors. If you believe you have low self-esteem, you may want to discuss this with a therapist and work on improving it. Building self-worth means accepting yourself as you are rather than looking for a new body or personality. Value who you are, and stop thinking in terms of, "If only . . . ." List your positive traits, and emphasize them to yourself. Stop the negative self-talk that can make you feel like a failure.

Talk About Your Feelings

Psychologists also recommend improving one's expression of feelings as another way to resist disordered eating. Sometimes overeating is a way of dealing with feelings that you do not want to face. In that case, food becomes a substitute for dealing with the real issue and does not solve the problem. Learn that it is safe and sane to talk about your feelings, even if they are not always positive.

WHAT FRIENDS CAN DO

Disordered eating behavior can be linked to perceptions and pressures from your peer group. Fitting in may mean doing something you do not want to do, such as developing disordered eating in order to be thin. It takes a lot of personal strength to resist the peer group's message, because all adolescents are struggling for acceptance while trying to establish independence from their parents.

On the other hand, peer groups can work to protect their members and to fight the triad. Peer groups have been formed in high schools, colleges, and among coworkers to help develop skills and healthy behaviors. Some well-known groups include Alateen (for teenagers affected by alcoholism), and Athletes in Action.

Peer education programs work to help women develop positive body images and resist pressures toward disordered eating. At Duke University, a campus organization called ESTEEM (Educational Support to Eliminate Eating Misconceptions) provides peer support and educational programs to the entire campus community. Trained peer educators lead seminars challenging the portrayal of women in the media, and they offer support to women struggling with weight issues. Such programs can change the entire social environment in a college or high school campus by actively striving to inform the community about eating disorders.

In the athletic realm, support groups have been formed to help women learn about the female athlete triad and develop their own methods for dealing with weight pressures. At UCLA, gymnasts formed a group to address weight issues and support each other in dealing with disordered eating. Working with nutritionists, psychologists, and medical professionals, they met regularly to problem solve. They developed strategies to resist overeating at holidays and to support each other during difficult training. The coach knew that these gymnasts were using medical professionals to advise them about weight control and felt relieved of this responsibility. He backed off on weigh-ins and body measurements. Everyone felt more relaxed and confident. Education and activism can be combined to defeat the female athlete triad. Women can be taught to observe and critique cultural messages and see how many images of themselves are unrealistic, unhealthy, and harmful.

WHAT FAMILIES CAN DO

There is no one family structure or upbringing that can prevent girls from developing the triad. But parents can do a lot to help their daughters navigate the difficult waters of adolescence and young adulthood, when most of the triad disorders begin. Much of what girls learn about their bodies and their health comes from early messages they get at home. A family that teaches moderation and respect for individuals and encourages open expressions of feelings can help immunize their daughters against disordered eating tendencies. Families can establish healthy eating patterns (including high levels of calcium intake during puberty for both boys and girls) based on sound nutritional goals, offering a wide variety of foods and regular meals. They can also discourage girls from dieting.

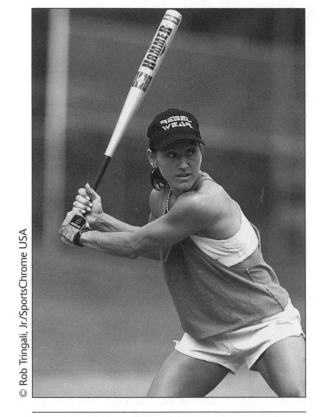

© Rob Tringali, Jr./SportsChrome USA

Friends and families can help young women develop
positive body images and healthy lifestyles.

Girls often learn dieting behavior first at home (often at a very
young age). If mothers or other family members diet or obsess about
weight, their daughters learn that this is expected and desirable behavior. Mothers should deal with their own weight and dieting issues by seeking professional help with a doctor, personal trainer, or
psychologist. By doing so, they can avoid inadvertently passing the
tendency to obsess about weight along to their daughters. Also, by
taking an active role to remedy their obsessions (and seeking professional help), they'll set a good example, and their daughters will see
that it is okay to seek help when you need it. Open lines of communication and acceptance between parents and daughters are helpful
in reducing the risk of eating disorders.

Family relationships need to grow and change as children develop
into adolescents. Adolescents struggle with independence, peer group
relationships, and changing bodies. It is a roller-coaster ride for the
entire family. Normal adolescents try out different lifestyles and begin

to establish their independence. Parents can help by keeping communication lines open and by actively listening and attempting to understand and accept these changes. Families that respect the individual, build self-worth, and instill a sense of a positive body image contribute to an adolescent's healthy outlook and positive self-esteem.

As girls begin puberty, they learn about their menstrual cycles from their mothers. Mothers can help daughters accept this change and learn basic information about the normal cycle, as well as managing cramps and PMS. They should take or encourage their daughters to go to the doctor if there is any change in menstrual cycle or if their daughters don't start puberty by age 14. Because preventing osteoporosis starts in childhood and adolescence, mothers and grandmothers can be role models, guiding the girls in their lives toward proper nutrition and exercise so that girls can build bone density and avoid this disease later in life.

A father's influence is critically important. Daughters are very sensitive to their fathers' messages about how they should look and act. Many girls have told me that their fathers accepted them the way they were and did not encourage weight loss. Their fathers' support made a great deal of difference when they were dealing with the ups and downs of adolescent body changes.

Families can also take an active role in educating themselves about the female athlete triad. Encourage open discussions about the triad and the factors leading toward it. Families can recognize and prepare their daughters for transition times like puberty and high school graduation. They can stay in touch and provide help, guidance, and support.

Guidelines for Families

- ◆ Establish and model healthy eating patterns.
- ◆ Ensure adequate calcium intake for each stage of life (see table 6.1).
- ◆ Avoid and discourage dieting behavior.
- ◆ Develop positive body image and sense of self-worth in children.
- ◆ Educate girls about the menstrual cycle and routine gynecological care.
- ◆ Mothers: Be a role model for osteoporosis prevention.
- ◆ Encourage open communication and self-expression.
- ◆ Accept the natural process of change, and continue to support daughters with interest, efforts to understand, and love.
- ◆ Fathers: Accept and love your daughters, wives, and mothers as they are. Avoid negative comments about weight and appearance.
- ◆ Seek family counseling if risk factors or warning signs of the triad disorders are present.

WHAT SCHOOLS AND
ORGANIZATIONS CAN DO

Educational efforts relating to healthy eating and exercise habits and ultimately the female athlete triad need to target individuals, professionals, and institutions. Education should begin early and should target both boys and girls. Starting in the first years of school, there should be a basic, core curriculum that covers nutrition, healthy exercise, the various body types, and the differences between boys' and girls' development. Educational exercises should emphasize acceptance of different body types and could include a critique of the impossible-to-attain media images of both women and men. Scare tactics are less effective than is focusing on positive messages about how proper nutrition fuels growth, physical activity, and academic performance. That kind of approach would help dispel the notion that food is an enemy and would promote it as a necessary fuel and a building block for success. Programs for youth and young adults emphasizing moderate exercise for lifelong fitness and health should be part of the curriculum so we can reduce the epidemic of childhood and adult obesity. The warning signs and dangers of disordered eating and the female athlete triad should be taught to both boys and girls.

We have gone to dorms, sororities, and conferences to lecture about the female athlete triad. There are numerous resources available for lecturing purposes, including videos and brochures from the NCAA and a slide series, video, and brochures from the American College of Sports Medicine (see resources section). One of the most effective presentations is to have a person who has experienced the triad (either as an athlete, coach, or professional) speak. Education done by and for peers is another excellent way to get the message across.

A national nonprofit organization, Eating Disorders Awareness and Prevention, has developed and distributed materials about preventing the first part of the triad, disordered eating. They sponsor a national Eating Disorders Awareness Week (usually in February) each year and provide materials for PTA, parents, professionals, and educators about community-based prevention methods.

Educational Methods of Preventing the Triad

◆ Add information about nutrition, exercise, body types, and building self-esteem to school curriculums.

◆ Educate about the warning signs and risks of the triad.

◆ Discourage dieting and educate about the risks of dieting.

◆ Dispel the myth that being thinner means being a better athlete.

◆ Critique media portrayals of men and women.

◆ Give lectures to groups about the triad.

◆ Participate in national Eating Disorders Prevention Week.

WHAT MEN CAN DO

Many men are unaware of how sensitive women are to comments about their weight and appearance. Most men have not experienced pressures to lose weight. They do not understand the frustration, despair, and sense of failure women feel when they are unsuccessful at reaching an impossible weight-loss goal. Often, men unconsciously contribute to the pressure with comments or attitudes. And although we have not focused much on men in this book, there are boys and men who develop serious eating disorders and osteoporosis. Education for men and boys needs to begin early and be a core part of prevention efforts for the triad. Educational topics could include female adolescent development, body composition, and prevention of harassment and violence toward women, as well as female athlete triad prevention. Both sexes can be educated together in programs that include respect for individuals of both sexes, and of all sizes, shapes, and colors.

If you are a father, brother, uncle, or coach, your role in helping healthy girls and women resist the triad is very important. Look closely at your attitudes about women in society at large. Most men have unconsciously formed attitudes toward women. Notice when you comment on weight or body fat around the women you care about. Are your comments positive? Practice evaluating women for characteristics other than their bodies. Tell the women in your life they look great the way they are. Tell them they don't need to lose any weight and you will love them no matter their weight. They will love you for it.

Education for men needs to include training that looks at attitudes about slimness and attractiveness. In the 1960s, we called this type of education consciousness raising. How might your attitudes and actions inadvertently put added pressure about weight loss on your daughters, sisters, girlfriends, or wives? Learn to listen to women's concerns, walk a few steps in their shoes, and discourage others from pressuring women to be unrealistically thin.

WHAT COACHES AND ATHLETIC DEPARTMENTS CAN DO

Since the female athlete triad was first recognized in athletic women, many prevention efforts have been directed at the athletic environment. One of the first steps is to make sure that policy in the athletic department does not mandate that people with eating disorders or the triad be excluded from team participation. These disorders are common, and if athletic departments seek to eliminate affected women, they will only drive them into hiding. An educated and enlightened athletic department will have resources in place to help these women and will ensure that coaches and training staff are educated about prevention and treatment of the triad.

Coaches should understand the basics of nutrition, the limitations of various methods of body composition testing (see chapter 1, pages 9 through 14), the differences in body types (see chapter 1, pages 18 through 22), and the importance of medical care. They should follow safe training practices and should know how to recognize and prevent overtraining. As mentioned previously, coaches should de-emphasize weight as an individual factor in performance and should emphasize attributes such as speed, strength, endurance, mental toughness, and power. Putting pressure on women to improve performance through weight loss alone brings out the negative issues associated with weight loss and creates a sense of frustration and failure.

Coaches should also avoid weigh-ins. If they do weigh-ins at all, they should not set weight goals for athletes without the input of the sports medicine staff. If there are indications for weight loss, these should be reviewed with the sports medicine staff using a program similar to the one developed by the University of Texas (see chapter 1, page 26).

Coaches should actively discourage unhealthy eating and dieting practices and should make sure that athletes come to practice and competition well nourished and hydrated. Coaches can be role models for healthy eating behavior when eating on the road and during long training sessions. Coaches working with women should have a basic understanding of women's developmental issues and the male/female differences in strength, body composition, and nutritional needs. Some of the training for coaches should sensitize them to women's issues about weight and comments about body fat. There is currently no universal coaching education program or coaching credential. Programs that offer coaching credentials should include education about all the topics just mentioned. Currently the Sanex WTA Tour has a coach's code of ethics (see resources).

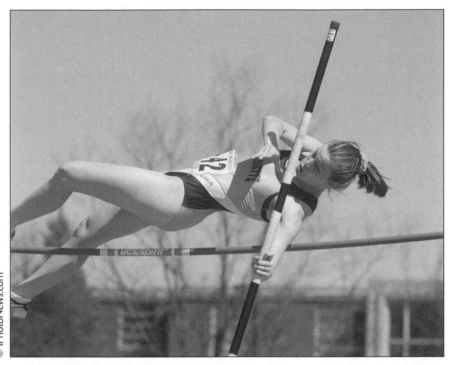

A knowledgeable and supportive coaching staff can help prevent and treat symptoms of the female athlete triad.

How Coaches Can Help

- ◆ Learn about basic nutrition, the limitations of various methods of body composition testing, different body types, and male/female differences.
- ◆ Develop connections in the sports medicine community to help you deal with weight issues, proper nutrition, and injury prevention.
- ◆ Follow training practices that are safe and that discourage development of the triad disorders.
- ◆ Recognize and avoid overtraining. Have your athletes keep a training log.
- ◆ Include a rest day, and vary the intensity of workouts so your athletes can recover.
- ◆ De-emphasize weight loss as the sole method of improving performance.
- ◆ Emphasize sport-related components of training, such as speed, power, endurance, and agility.

- ◆ Prohibit group weigh-ins.
- ◆ Discourage unhealthy eating and dieting practices.
- ◆ Be a role model for healthy eating behavior.
- ◆ Recognize the warning signs and risk factors for the female athlete triad.
- ◆ Promptly refer any athlete with menstrual cycle changes, weight issues, or injury.

It is our hope that everyone who reads even part of this book will be inspired to do something to prevent and fight the female athlete triad. If you have been affected in any way by these disorders, you know their serious nature and their ability to rob women of the joy of being their best. We must do all we can to prevent more women from being affected and from losing their health, the best years of their athletic careers, and even their lives. Perhaps you will be inspired not only to take on educational and prevention efforts but also to help research how to best prevent the triad. Take time now and make a list of several things you can and are willing to do to prevent the triad. Your time, thought, and effort will be worth it if you reach just one person.

We have spent several years and have worked with many wonderful, committed people in writing this book, in the hope that it will reach you. Now you can reach others. Please join us and many others in doing the work that must be done to recognize, prevent, and treat the female athlete triad. The next generation of women deserves to be too fit to quit rather than too thin to win.

References

American College of Sports Medicine. 1995. ACSM position stand on osteoporosis and exercise. *Medicine and Science in Sports and Exercise* 27(4):i-ix.

American Psychiatric Association. 1994. *Diagnostic and statistical manual of mental disorders,* 4th ed. Washington, DC: American Psychiatric Association.

Cates, S., and J. Steen. 1996. *Taking the disorder out of eating.* Chapel Hill, NC: Duke University.

Clark, N. 1997. *Nancy Clark's sports nutrition guidebook,* 2nd ed. Champaign, IL: Human Kinetics.

———. 1992. Women and weight: Making friends with Mother Nature. *The Physician and Sports Medicine* 20(3):41-42.

Drinkwater, B.L., K. Nilson, C.H. Chesnut III, W.J. Bremner, S. Shainholtz, and M.B. Southworth. 1984. Bone mineral content of amenorrheic and eumenorrheic athletes. *New England Journal of Medicine* 311(5):277-281.

Drinkwater, B.L., B. Bruemner, and C.H. Chesnut III. 1990. Menstrual history as a determinant of current bone density in young athletes. *Journal of the American Medical Association* 263(4):545-548.

Dueck, C.A., K.S. Matt, M.M. Manore, and J.S. Skinner. 1996. Treatment of athletic amenorrhea with a diet and training intervention program. *International Journal of Sport Nutrition* 6:24-40.

Grigg, M. 1996. Disordered eating and unhealthy weight reduction practices among adolescent females. *Preventive Medicine* 25(6):748-756.

International Tennis Federation. 1998. ITF's code of ethics for coaches. *ITF Coaches Review* 16:14-15.

Johnson, C., P.S. Powers, and R. Dick. 1999. Athletes and eating disorders: The National Collegiate Athletic Association study. *International Journal of Eating Disorders* 26(2):179-188.

Keys, A., et al. 1950. *The biology of human starvation.* Minneapolis: University of Minnesota Press.

Locke, R.J., and M.P. Warren. 2000. How to prevent bone loss in women with hypothalamic amenorrhea. *Women's Health in Primary Care* 3(4):270-278.

Lohman, T.G., L. Houtkooper, and S.B. Going. 1997. Body fat measurement goes high-tech. *ACSM's Health and Fitness Journal* 1(1): 33-34.

Meyer, J.E., J.M. Leiman, N. Rothschild, and M. Falik. 1999. *Improving the health of adolescent girls.* New York: The Commonwealth Fund Commission on Women's Health.

Myburgh, K.H., J. Hutchins, A.B. Fataar, S.F. Hough, and T.D. Noakes. 1990. Low bone density is an etiologic factor for stress fractures in athletes. *Annals of Internal Medicine* 113(10):754-759.

Myburgh, K.H., et al. 1992. Are risk factors for menstrual dysfunction cumulative? *Physician and Sportsmedicine* 20(4):114-125.

Otis, C. L. 1992. Exercise associated amenorrhea. *Clinical Sports Medicine* 11(2):351-362.

Otis C.L., B.L. Drinkwater, M. Johnson, A. Loucks, and J.H. Wilmore. 1997. ACSM position stand on the female athlete triad. *Medicine and Science in Sport and Exercise* 29(5)i-ix.

Rosen, L.W., et al. 1986. Pathogenic weight-control behavior in female athletes. *Physician and Sportsmedicine* 1479-1486.

Ryan, R. 1992. Management of eating problems in athletic settings. In *Eating, Body Weight and Performance in Athletes: Disorders of Modern Society.* Ed. K.D. Brownell, J. Rodin, and J.H. Wilmore. Philadelphia: Lea and Febiger, 344-360.

Sizer, F., and E. Whitney. 2000. *Nutrition concepts and controversies,* 8th ed. Belmont: CA: Thomson Learning.

Solin, S. 1997. Do you have a healthy body image? *Fitness* October: 94-97.

Sundgot-Borgen, J. 1994. Risk and trigger factors for the development of eating disorders in female elite athletes. *Medicine and Science in Sport and Exercise* 26:414-419.

Warren, M.P., J. Brooks-Gunn, L.H. Hamilton, L. Fiske Warren, and W.G. Hamilton. 1986. Scoliosis and fractures in young ballet dancers: Relation to delayed menarche and secondary amenorrhea. *New England Journal of Medicine* 314:1348-1353.

Wasnich, R.D. 1991. "Bone mass measurements in diagnosis and assessment of therapy," *American Journal of Medicine* 91(5B):54S-58S.

Wells, C. 1991. *Women, sport, and performance,* 2nd ed. Champaign, IL: Human Kinetics.

Wilmore, J., and D. Costill. 1999. *Physiology of sport and exercise,* 2nd ed. Champaign, IL: Human Kinetics.

Resources

Books

Agostini, R. 1994. *Medical and orthopedic issues of active and athletic women.* Philadelphia: Hanley and Belfus.

Brownell, K.D., J. Rodin, and J.H. Wilmore, eds. 1992. *Eating, body weight, and performance in athletes.* Philadelphia: Lea and Febiger.

Freedman, R. 1988. *Body love: Learning to like our looks and ourselves.* Carlsbad, CA: Gürze Books.

Gaesser, G. 1996. *Big fat lies: The truth about your weight and your health.* New York: Fawcett Columbine.

Goodman, L. 1992. *Is your child dying to be thin? A workbook for parents and family members on eating disorders.* Pittsburgh: Dorrance.

Hall, L. 1993. *Full lives: Women who have freed themselves from food and weight obsessions.* Carlsbad, CA: Gürze Books.

Lutter, J.M. 1998. *Of heroes, hope and level playing fields.* St. Paul: Melpomene.

Lutter, J.M., and L. Jaffee. 1996. *The bodywise woman.* Champaign, IL: Human Kinetics.

Otis, C.L., and R. Goldingay. 1989. *Campus health guide: The college students' handbook for healthy living.* New York: The College Board.

Rodin, J. 1993. *Body traps: Breaking the binds that keep you from feeling good about yourself.* New York: Morrow.

Thompson, R.A., and R.T. Sherman. 1992. *Helping athletes with eating disorders.* Champaign, IL: Human Kinetics.

Associations

American Anorexia Bulimia Association, Inc. (AABA), 165 West 46th Street, Suite 1108, New York, NY 10036; call 212-575-6200; **www.aabainc.org.** Offers public information, East Coast treatment referrals, support groups, speakers, educational programs, professional training.

American Dietetic Association (ADA), 216 West Jackson Boulevard, Chicago, IL 60606; call 312-899-0040 or 800-366-1655; **www.eatright.org.** In addition to its excellent Web site, the ADA offers a hotline that allows you to speak to a licensed dietitian and provides the names of licensed dietitians for specific locations.

Anorexia Nervosa and Related Eating Disorders (ANRED), Box 5102, Eugene, OR 97405; call 541-344-1144; **www.anred.com.** Offers some free information on its Web site and works in association with EDAP.

Eating Disorders Awareness and Prevention (EDAP), 603 Stewart Street, Suite 803, Seattle, WA 98101; call 206-382-3587 or 800-931-2237; **www.edap.org.** Sponsors National Eating Disorders Awareness Week in February. Offers health care professionals, educators, and the public prevention and awareness information, educational programs, videos, curricula, a newsletter, conferences, workshops, and a national speakers bureau. Also provides a toll-free information and resource line.

National Association of Anorexia and Associated Disorders (ANAD), Box 7, Highland Park, IL 60035; **www.anad.org.** ANAD is a nonprofit organization that focuses on helping eating disorder victims and their families. In addition to its free hotline counseling (847-831-3438), ANAD operates an international network of support groups for sufferers and families and offers referrals to health care professionals who treat eating disorders. ANAD also publishes a national quarterly newsletter to its members for a $25.00 annual contribution and will mail information packets customized to individual needs on request.

The National Eating Disorders Information Centre (NEDIC), CW 1-211, 200 Elizabeth Street, Toronto, Ontario M5G 2C4 Canada; call 416-340-4156; **www.nedic.on.ca.** NEDIC provides information and resources on eating disorders and food and weight preoccupation, a Canada-wide database of intervention resources, and Canadian Eating Disorders Awareness Week.

National Institutes of Health Osteoporosis and Related Bone Diseases~National Resource Center (NIH ORBD~NRC), 1232 22nd St. NW, Washington, DC 20037-1292; call 202-223-0344 or 800-624-BONE; **www.osteo.org.** NIH ORBD~NRC provides a link between current resources and the health professionals, patients, and public who are trying to locate these resources.

National Osteoporosis Foundation (NOF), 1232 22nd Street NW, Washington, DC 20037-1292; call 202-223-2226 or 800-400-1079; **www.nof.org.** The most well-known source for osteoporosis information.

Overeaters Anonymous (OA), P.O. Box 44020, Rio Rancho, NM 87174-4020; call 505-891-2664; **www.oa.org.** A nationwide 12-step self-help fellowship offering free local meetings listed in the white pages under Overeaters Anonymous.

Sanex WTA Tour, 133 1st Street NE, St. Petersburg, FL 33701; **www.sanexwta.com.** The Web site has information on the Coach's Code of Ethics and health information for active women.

Other Resources

Education, Training, Research (ETR) Associates provides a handbook on body image. ETR Associates, PO Box 1830, Santa Cruz, CA; call 800-321-4407; **www.etr.org.**

Gürze Books, Eating Disorder Resources, Box 2238, Carlsbad, CA 92018; call 800-756-7533; **www.gurze.com.** Gürze specializes in eating disorders education and publications.

Healthy Weight Network, 402 South 14th Street, Hettinger, ND 58639; call 701-567-2646; **www.healthyweight.net.** You'll find news releases and ready-to-print handouts and posters.

Nutrition and Eating Disorders Video Series. Produced by the National Collegiate Athletic Association (NCAA). Available through Karol Media, 350 North Pennsylvania Ave. P.O. Box 7600, Wilkes-Barre, PA 18773-7600; call 800-884-0555; **www. karolmedia.com.** This three-video series (48 minutes) covers the problems created by losing weight without the proper nutrition; the consequences of eating disorders; and what coaches, teachers, and others can do to help the student-athlete. Titles include *Afraid to Eat: Eating Disorders and the Student-Athlete*; *Out of Balance: Nutrition and Weight*; and *Eating Disorders: What Can You Do?* A set of printed materials suitable for copying accompanies the series. Cost: $39.95, plus $5.00 shipping and handling.

Real Women Project. Web site: **www.realwomenproject.com.** "Real Women" is a series of 13 small, bronze sculptures and poems portraying women of diverse sizes, shapes, and cultures spanning eight decades of life.

Something Fishy Web site on Eating Disorders at **www.somethingfishy.org.** This page provides numerous links and extensive information about eating disorders and body image issues.

National Federation of State High School Associations TARGET Program, 690 W. Washington St., Indianapolis, IN 46204; 317-972-6900. Web site: **www.nfhs.org.** NFHS has the following brochure available: *Preseason Meeting Handbook.* Cost: $4.95, plus $4.00 shipping and handling. This 24-page publication guides coaches, activity sponsors, and athletic directors through the preseason meeting process. The preseason meeting provides an excellent forum to discuss healthy lifestyle issues such as proper nutrition and prevention of disordered eating.

Index

Note: Page numbers in *italics* refer to figures; those in **boldface** refer to tables.

About The Authors

As physician for the UCLA Student Health Services, **Carol L. Otis, MD**, has worked with many women, seeing firsthand the devastating effects of the triad. She received her medical degree from the University of Southern California and currently serves as the chief medical advisor for the Women's Professional Tennis (Sanex WTA Tour). Dr. Otis was also a former assistant team physician for the UCLA varsity athletic teams and adjunct assistant clinical professor in UCLA's Division of Internal Medicine.

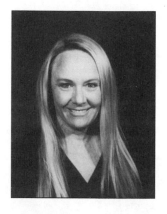

Dr. Otis has worked with athletes in numerous sports, acting as physician for the Boston Marathon, Ironman World Championship Triathlon, gymnastics teams at the 1984 Olympic Games in Los Angeles, and for the U.S. Olympic Track and Field Trials. She's worked to draw awareness to female athlete issues through her position as former chairperson of the Strategic Health Initiative for Women for the American College of Sports Medicine, as well as her work with the USTA Sports Science Committee and ITF Medical Commission. Dr. Otis also maintains an extensive lecturing schedule, has published many research studies and articles on women in sports, and has appeared on the *Today Show* to discuss female athletes and amenorrhea. She and coauthor Roger Goldingay are married and live in Los Angeles, California. They can be contacted through their Web site **www.sportsdoctor.com**.

Roger Goldingay, a former professional soccer player, is presently a Web designer, writer, and photographer. With his wife, Dr. Carol L. Otis, he coauthored *Campus Health Guide* (College Board, 1989) as well as monthly columns for *Shape* and *Women's Sport & Fitness*. His own writing has appeared in many magazines, including *Runner's World, Men's Fitness,* and *Sports Medicine Digest*.

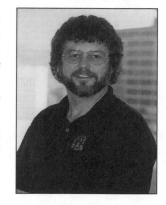